# Empty Your Stress Bucket

## ...and keep it empty for life

# Gin Lalli

tonic titles

Published in 2021 by Tonic Titles

Copyright © Gin Lalli 2021

Gin Lalli has asserted her right to be identified as the author of this Work
in accordance with the Copyright, Designs and Patents Act 1988

ISBN Paperback: 978-1-7399775-0-4
Ebook: 978-1-7399775-1-1

All rights reserved. No part of this publication may be reproduced,
stored in a retrieval system, or transmitted in any form or by any means,
electronic, mechanical, photocopying, recording or otherwise, without the
prior permission of the copyright owner.

A CIP catalogue copy of this book can be found in the British Library.

Published with the help of Indie Authors World
www.indieauthorsworld.com

IndieAuthors
World

For Dad, who has taught me how to stay in Charhdi Kala (eternal optimism and joy) to keep the stress bucket empty.

## Acknowledgements.

No book is really written by one person, it may have been me sitting here typing away for months on end but it wouldn't have been at all possible without support

So....

Anil Sekhari and "the management committee" - can you get off my case now please! At least for a few weeks anyway!

David Newton and CPHT Leeds – LS1 were the original and the best were we not? In particular 2 fantastic tutors Jenny Mellenchip and Cathy Eland – you made learning fun! Special mention to Jenny Mellenchip for continued mentorship to this day and reading of drafts.

Kim MacLeod and Indie Authors World thanks for getting me over the line.

Michael Heppell, and the first Write That Book Masterclass – I got there in the end! The journey was immense! Thank you so much for your guidance and encouragement.

Mike Guard, you gave me the right nudge at the right time – thank you.

Alan Smith and the Action Coach group in Edinburgh – what a motivational team you all are. That talk at Action Club gave me the biggest boost ever – you'll never know. (Nicholas Blurton – I use your 'stress skip' quote to this day!)

Julie Diver at 39Steps for my illustrations – your talent and creativity amaze me with every piece of artwork that drops into my inbox #JulieDoodles

Squad Rants and Goals – you know who you are and nothing needs saying!

Sandra Benn and Sandy Cullen, 2 mentors and friends that are always there for me. I know you'll say it's nothing but it's loads to me. How will I ever repay you?

Claire Watson for actually making me enjoy having my photograph taken

Denise Strohsahl of Sandstonecastles Marketing – how you put up with me I will never know but I am eternally grateful "Step away from that shiny new thing, Gin!"

Hazel Johnstone – my 1-woman PR machine who does not realise she is my 1-woman PR machine!

Tom, Maria, Colette and the whole gang at Healthy Life Centre. I had so much to learn in the beginning and your encouragement, support and enthusiasm made it all a joy!

And finally, to each and every one of my clients, past, present and future. Your commitment to change and your absolute resolve to empty your stress bucket inspires me every single time – I learn more from you than you do from me. It has been a privilege to work with you towards your goals and more. May your bucket remain empty and your sleep plentiful.

# Introduction

Why do some people cope with life's challenges and others don't?

Why do we have this crisis in mental health?

No-one has lived a perfect life without any stress. Everyone is affected by bereavement, family strain, financial pressures, career issues...the list goes on. There is also no pattern to show that some people are affected more than others. Nothing related to gender, age or race to say *clearly* that a certain demographic is significantly more susceptible to poor mental health.

I love the fact we are beginning to scratch the surface to be more open and talk about things like depression and anxiety which were previously kept behind closed doors. Mental health awareness is a great movement and I don't want to take anything away from it. We have never been more aware of mental health issues than we are right now.

But... The time has come for action. Awareness isn't enough.

It frustrates me that we have not yet found something to help. With such huge advances in medicine and science why have we not yet found 'the cure'? If anything, it seems that mental illness is on the rise.

So where do we begin?

We need to study those who cope really well with life's challenges. Those who can manage their stress, create resilience and come out the other side, plodding on, determined and strong, eventually feeling happy and fulfilled once more. Surely life is happening to all of us and we all have to face the many challenges that arise along the way. People with good mental health have not led fairy-tale lives, yet they have a certain resilience that keeps them going even when they don't feel like it.

What is it that makes us different from other animals that our emotions can overwhelm us? That we can be consumed by those feelings so completely?

I strongly believe that knowledge is power and having an understanding of where these feelings come from is a huge step in making progress going forward.

And although we can't all have a degree in biomedical science or a doctorate in human anatomy, basic knowledge of the brain can be very valuable in beginning to understand the symptoms of mental illness.

Understanding where those feelings of anxiety, depression and anger come from makes a huge difference in comprehending ourselves as human beings with the vast array of feelings and emotions we possess.

Have you ever felt anxious going into a meeting or before a presentation? Have you ever felt sad, even depressed, after a bereavement? Have you ever felt angry with road rage or something that's really annoyed you?

These are all normal emotions and if you have ever felt anxious, angry or depressed, then well done, your brain is working just fine. Short bursts of negative emotions are only natural and often drive us to make positive change. The mind and body are well-equipped for this. But if those feelings consume you to such an extent that they affect your everyday life then something needs to be done. Because how long can this carry on?

Stress is a normal part of life and it should be seen that way. Those feelings arising from stress can be managed and overcome. Short bouts of stress are quite normal and something we are biologically programmed to deal with, in fact, the human spirit can be surprisingly robust; however, long-term stress can not only cause mental issues but can also affect you physically. Increased blood pressure, heart disease, type 2 diabetes are all known as a lifestyle diseases and are on the rise.

Before I qualified as a psychotherapist, I had a very fulfilling career as an optometrist. I loved the work and meeting many people with their different stories fascinated me. I quickly came to realise that everyone has a story and my clinic would often fall behind as I loved to hear about their lives. Having a natural propensity to chat, I never found this difficult and I would revel in talking to people at length. People who had fought in wars and travelled, people with interesting jobs and unusual family backgrounds.

Now we didn't start talking about life randomly. Optometrists always have to check a patient's medical background, to consider if there will be ocular side effects from general health issues or medication. Having an eye examination is also a good general health check, as we can often pick up signs of things like high blood pressure or type 2 diabetes. I found over the years I was doing this more often; referring people to their GP for a blood pressure check when I saw convoluted blood vessels at the back of the eye, or if there were a few tiny haemorrhages on the retina I would advise a blood-glucose test with their practice nurse as soon as possible.

This is where the storytelling would begin. Comments such as: 'I bet my blood pressure is high, I've not had an easy time of it' or 'I knew this would happen, I don't look after myself properly' were all too prevalent. As I got talking to these people in a bit more detail, it was surprising how comfortable they were telling me their stories. Maybe taking those few moments with a professional who was prepared to listen made them take stock and assess how they had got to this juncture. After hearing many life experiences from so many different people, there was always one underlying cause: stress.

Stress of all types and of varying degrees. A bereavement or huge loss years earlier that someone had not come to terms with. Maybe ongoing family or financial pressures were keeping someone awake at night. Anger and frustration caused by a stressful work environment. Over a prolonged period of time this was now affecting someone's physical health.

I remember once seeing an eighteen-year-old on anti-depressants. After chatting for a while, they told me they were getting no other support at all. They weren't being shown any life skills or supported in other ways that would help them manage or cope in the future. These 'magic' pills were to solve this problem. An eighteen-year-old with their whole life ahead of them? How was that the solution? I was becoming very disheartened at the prevalence of mental health issues.

I didn't always see people who were sick though. Regular eye exams are always good and if you need to wear spectacles, like me, they are part of your regular routine. So, it was always nice to see people who said 'no, nothing' when I asked 'are you on any medication?' This was always most surprising when I saw someone elderly. I loved seeing someone of mature years, not only because they liked to chat, but because they always had a fascinating story to tell and I loved to hear any advice they shared.

I would ask them what it was that made them so healthy, what was their secret? After humbly saying that it wasn't much at all, they went on to tell me of a life of stress, of challenges with family, bereavements, and maybe a difficult work life. It was the same story as those people who were now physically sick. The only difference was that these people had something I couldn't quite put my finger on. This sort of resilience or resolve to meet life's challenges head on. To accept what they could not control, and do what they could with the rest. To make the most of life, whatever cards they had been dealt. I was in awe of these people. Their tenacity, the spirit with which they were tackling all of life's challenges. It made me think that we need to study these people more. Instead of examining the mechanics of depression or the symptoms of anxiety we should be looking for the solution to these issues instead. What is going on inside determined people that we can all learn from? Could knowing that help that eighteen-year-old on antidepressants? It seemed to me that these people held the 'cure' for mental health and yet they could not explain what it was.

Having a background in science meant that there was only one way for me to understand this – get the facts around it. So, there was only one thing for it; I had to study the brain!

What is going on inside that fascinating organ that we all possess but differs from one person to another?

Of the many forms of therapy and counselling I researched, solution-focused therapy appealed to me the most. It spoke my language – the science of brain function – seeing as I'd already studied about a third of the brain known as the visual cortex. It also appealed to me personally as it is focused on looking forward rather than backwards. To stop going over the past, make the most of the present and use that to create change for the future.

In this book I aim to help you understand the science of stress, how it originates in the brain and what you can do to empty your stress bucket. I try to impart my knowledge, what I have come to learn through working with people to change their lives, from talking to family, friends and clients who have coped and managed through some extraordinary challenges, and the vast amount taught to me by some amazing tutors. I hope what you read here will help you to overcome anxiety and stress-related issues like depression, phobias, fears, lack of motivation, low self-esteem and lack of confidence, so that you can live a long, healthy and happy life.

## Brain Basics

L et's look at the brain.

Right now, you're using the intelligent part of your brain to read this – the vast resource of all that learning you did as a child that you've now programmed yourself to be able to read without even thinking about it. This is the part of the brain that you know as being YOU. It's your consciousness, the objective and rational part of your brain. This part of the brain allows us to drive, use computers and mobile phones. In fact, this is the part of the brain you use to analyse a situation, assess it carefully, then come up with the right answer to take some action. So, it's generally quite positive. Because it's attached to all your intelligent resources I 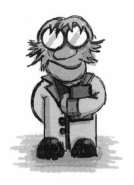 call it the **intelligent brain** – if you want to be fancy, it's your left prefrontal cortex but let's keep it simple and call it the intelligent brain for now.

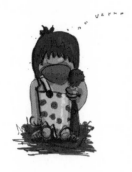

Now there's another part of your brain I want to talk about – the original, primitive part of your brain. You'll know this part of your brain as it's commonly called the 'fight or flight' response, medically known as the amygdala. This part of the brain is our survival response from caveman days and it has served us well over time. I'll call this part of the brain the **primitive brain**.

So how do these two parts of the brain work together?

Imagine if you will, that you looked up from reading right now and saw a massive polar bear coming towards you – what would happen?

Your stress levels would shoot up instantly, you would lose the intellectual control you had while reading and your primitive brain would kick into gear straight away.

Your heart would start pumping to get the oxygen flowing quickly to your muscles so you could make a run for it, you'd breathe a lot faster, you'd go all sweaty and your guts would churn – in fact you'd probably have a full-blown panic attack, you'd scream the place down while running as fast as your little legs could carry you.

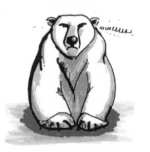

And that's fantastic – get away from that polar bear and survive – fight or flight – you don't want to die! In any case, fight might be the riskier option, it may be better to run away (flight) instead.

But it's much the same in life – as your stress levels rise you begin to lose the intellectual control from the intelligent brain and the primitive brain steps in to take over.

Your stress levels can rise gradually over time. You don't need a sudden event to make that happen. A sudden traumatic event will naturally raise your stress levels. But often you can't pinpoint it to one specific event, maybe just a multitude of life's stresses, building up over days, months and years.

The primitive brain senses danger ahead, so takes over to go into survival mode. It's a safety mechanism.

The primitive brain has three opt-out clauses and we are all pre-programmed with these.

They are:

depression

anxiety

anger

Let's look at these individually in more detail.

## Caveman Theory

If your mind, as a whole, senses some sort of danger ahead, your primitive brain will step in, take over and go into one of these opt-out clauses of depression, anxiety and anger, or even a combination of all three. (Yes, you can actually be depressed, angry and anxious all at the same time).

If we look back through evolution, we can clearly see the reason why we have these three responses.

Imagine our caveman ancestors, looking out of the cave one day and seeing it all snowed under. They would think *Forget this, I'm not going out hunting and gathering today. I'll just retreat back into my cave, pull the rug over my head and wait until this situation passes!* And that would have been a perfectly appropriate survival response under those circumstances. Except we don't live like that any more. We've taken that primitive response and translated it into modern day symptoms of depression.

You can't get out of bed, or get motivated to do things. You want to hide away from the world and sleep the day away. When we're depressed, we lack motivation to do even the simplest of tasks.

Imagine the caveman out hunting and gathering in the wild. They had to be alert for danger all the time. Another tribe or animal could be just around the corner ready to attack. We don't live like that any more, but we've taken that natural survival response and we now call it anxiety.

We are worried about what might happen and concerned for the dangers that may be out there. You may be constantly worried about your family, or issues at work. You are concerned and overthink about your future prospects. You wonder how you will ever get through the day with all the challenges that lie ahead.

And anger... Well, that's simply a primitive response to fear. If the poor caveman was ever attacked, what did they do to scare that tribe or animal away? They screamed and shouted, grinned and bared their teeth, made themselves bigger by flailing their arms about to scare that danger away – and these days when we see that in someone, we say they've got anger management issues. Maybe you're snapping at people for no obvious reason, or feeling argumentative all the time. Road rage is a perfect example of this.

Look a little closer.

Remember I said the primitive brain was the fight or flight part?

Well…

anger is fight,

anxiety is flight

and depression is freeze

– we should actually call it 'fight, flight or freeze.'

Generalised anxiety disorders, clinical depression and anger management issues don't simply occur overnight though. The response can be short and sharp, but once you get 'emotionally hijacked' by the primitive brain it is all consuming.

Early signs of the anger response (fight) can be feeling irritable, grumpy or having a short temper. Feeling slightly anxious (flight) initially shows up as constant worry, fear and being overly pessimistic. And depression symptoms can first appear as low mood, a lack of motivation and procrastination; it's too dangerous to come out of your 'cave'. Try to spot the signs early on, don't let it build up so it overpowers you completely because that's when you lose control.

One for the computer geeks:

I often use this example to help people understand how the brain has evolved though time.

Imagine your brain as a computer. The primitive brain is very old hardware that has not had an upgrade for centuries. Instead of upgrading and developing that part of the computer, a whole load of new software in the form of the intelligent brain has been attached to it instead. This new software is constantly getting upgraded and monitored (and getting even larger). The old hardware is still there. But now there is a conflict between the old out-of-date hardware and the new sophisticated software… The whole computer is not working as efficiently as it could, especially when the old hardware is just as powerful as it ever was.

Can you see how these once very useful survival responses really do not serve us well in modern times? The fight response is now seen as anger management issues, the flight response is now generalised anxiety disorder and the prolonged freeze response is clinical depression.

There are a few more things you should know about the primitive brain.

### The primitive brain is negative

It's not only negative but it is *extremely* negative and it goes to the extreme negative very quickly.

Imagine if you saw that polar bear – you wouldn't take your time to weigh up and assess the situation for some positive possibilities. You wouldn't think *oh, hang on a minute, this might be a vegetarian polar bear here – it might not eat me today! I might be alright!*

In order to survive, in a split second, you would think *aaaaagh, I'm gonna die!* and that would make you immediately run as fast as you could to escape the danger.

And so it is in life.

If the primitive brain has kicked in, you will catastrophise immediately, thinking of the worst-case scenario to ensure you take the right action.

However, the worst-case scenario is often so far focused into the future that it creates immediate anxiety, or causes you to buckle under the depression. Despite the fact that it's unlikely to happen, your primitive brain has now taken over so there is no reasoning with it – it's gone into survival mode.

Catastrophising, one of the biggest causes of mental ill health, is when you assume that the worst will happen. Often, it involves believing that you're in a worse situation than you really are or exaggerating the difficulties you face. For example, someone might worry that they'll fail an exam. If they fail that exam, it means they won't get the qualification they need. Their imagination now begins to run away with that thought very quickly. Well, if they don't get qualified, they'll never be a success in life, never get the house/car/relationship they want – they're going to die! (That example might be a bit extreme and dramatic but it does happen). This negative spiral of thinking is catastrophising and you may have found yourself doing that with only the smallest trigger to begin with.

It can also become very draining, constantly considering everything that might go wrong when in reality it may never happen. Most of the things we worry about don't ever actually occur, or at least they never occur in the way we had imagined. It can take up a lot of time and energy in your 'headspace' to catastrophise.

### The primitive brain is obsessional

If there was a polar bear outside it would be a good idea to keep a check on it, wouldn't it?

Is it still there?

Has it gone yet?

You shouldn't take your eyes off it; it could attack you when you aren't looking, so keep your eyes fixed on it.

These days we've found other things to 'keep a check on'. Once again, we've taken that primitive survival response and translated it to modern times.

Maybe you keep checking your phone for no reason at all.

You keep checking you've locked the door, switches are off, or you've checked twenty times you've got your passports and tickets before you leave to travel.

Maybe you have obsessive and repetitive thoughts. Repeating the same old scenarios in your head over and over again. Or maybe thinking about the same problem or same issue with no relief at all.

In severe cases you can even develop OCD (obsessive compulsive disorder).

It makes sense to the primitive brain to get obsessed with checking the locks as it helps you to feel safe. By developing an OCD, it makes you feel like you're in control, it alleviates the symptoms of anxiety for merely a moment.

Your mind looks for something to get obsessional about to keep you safe.

## The primitive brain is vigilant

If there's one polar bear, well it would be a good idea to keep an eye out for more polar bears... There could be another one up the road and two more round the corner! Stay alert.

Translating that response to modern times – we are vigilant about the next problem to occur in our life.

*Well, if this doesn't work, I bet the next thing I do won't work either and I'll never manage that whole thing – it will all go wrong I just know it!*

That constant state of high alert is pure anxiety in itself.

An interesting point to note here is the vigilance you may feel when you want to go to sleep.

You know, those racing thoughts and very active mind that doesn't 'switch off'?

If you are stressed and your mind senses danger, the primitive, survival response will NOT let you sleep. Why would it? A polar bear might attack. You need to keep your defences up and stay alert – the last thing you should be doing is sleeping.

You need to learn to relax, you need to use your intelligent brain to look at the situation more objectively – you are safe and cosy in your bed – it's time to sleep, it's time to rest.

Any slight noise makes you jump, you're wary and cautious all the time. This takes up a lot of energy and you can become physically exhausted.

Therefore, that constant state of vigilance, and even hyper-vigilance, is really not serving us well now.

**

*Jennifer's story*

As I help people with insomnia and sleep issues, I am often asked if I can help someone to stop snoring – the request will come from the person being disturbed by the snoring (would they be called the snoree???) not the snorer.

Jennifer came to see me as her partner was snoring so loudly, she thought they would have to end their otherwise very happy fifteen-year marriage. As Jennifer learned that I focused a lot of my therapy on the value of sleep, she asked me if it would be okay to give my details to her husband and could I have a chat with him to convince him to come and see me. She felt he was probably not getting a good night's sleep himself, and the knock-on effect was really taking its toll on her. If solution-focused therapy could stop him snoring then Jennifer would be so happy.

I took some time to chat with Jennifer and found out that she had a very stressful role at work. She had recently been promoted and, although she enjoyed the challenge, she was concerned that she was not yet performing to her best and was worried she would be seen as a bit of an imposter. She had also recently been taking care of one of her parents who needed frequent visits to the hospital for some treatment (often a 100-mile round trip). She was exhausted and naturally concerned about this. It was clear to me that Jennifer's stress bucket was filling up fast.

I explained to her that, although I would love to chat with her husband, it was really up to him. It seemed likely that Jennifer would benefit from my help more than her husband. He had not yet realised the impact it was having on Jennifer. I felt that it would be best for Jennifer to come and see me for a course of sessions first and I explained why;

Her husband was having a lovely night's sleep and happily dreaming away in the land of nod, but she was being kept awake and no doubt the lack of sleep was adding to her already quite high stress levels. ANY noise, from a dripping tap to snoring hubby, felt so loud that Jennifer was being disturbed; she was being vigilant. And where does vigilance come from? The primitive brain, where anxiety and depression are opt-out clauses. If there really was a polar bear, the last thing Jennifer should do is sleep. She had tuned in to her danger.

Once we worked on emptying her stress bucket, her vigilance dropped and she was able to relax, getting a good night's sleep even with hubby snoring away.

> Jennifer learned that you should be able to relax, and even sleep, with normal everyday sounds around you. These noises are not dangers any more, you know that from your intelligent brain. But if you're functioning from your primitive brain, all you can think is *polar bear ahead! Danger! Do not sleep!*

**\*\***

We are born with only two fears: falling and noise. These are our in-built survival responses. Therefore, noise is one of the biggest triggers for stress and anxiety. This is why when we are stressed and anxious, we often find that even music can be very jarring. If we empty the stress bucket we can begin to enjoy those lovely sounds again. You can literally gauge how full your stress bucket is by any irrational responses to everyday sounds.

## The primitive brain is not creative

If yesterday you saw a polar bear and you ran in a certain direction and survived, you'd program yourself with that behaviour and ensure you do the exact same thing again the next time you see a polar bear. A brilliant survival response but not so good in modern times.

The primitive brain stores that survival response for the next, and every, time you feel like that again. It won't explore other options. Because the primitive brain is not an intellect it will not rationalise the situation, it needs to react immediately and swiftly to save you.

Basically, you get a very fixed mindset. (It's in the intelligent brain that you have more of a creative, growth mindset).

You will repeat the same behaviours over and over again because in your primitive brain you think it works.

The very first time you were stressed how did you react? Did you reach for a bottle of wine? Or did you storm off feeling really angry? Whatever you did, that very first time you did it you may have got some sort of feeling of relief from the stress. Well, you'll now do that each and every time you need to react to a stressful situation. It's your default response now. Intelligently, you know you want to break this habit but you're now consumed by the primitive brain so there is only one way to react.

This sort of 'emotional hijacking' becomes an ever-vicious circle. You cannot think logically when you perceive a threat, therefore your choices of how to behave are very limited. Your brain creates more demands on you and more absolute and finite responses. Words such as 'must', 'should', 'always', and 'never' become the default of the mind's vocabulary. This in turn creates an increased sense of threat…and so the cycle continues.

Can you see that the primitive brain, that served us so well through caveman times, is not serving us so well in modern times ? We have taken the polar bear response and now we see metaphorical polar bears in our lives.

Can you think of people or situations that have become your new polar bear? Maybe it's an overflowing email inbox, the pressures put on you by your boss, or an ever-demanding family life. However, we need to learn to rationalise these thoughts and feelings. Although these things may be stressful, they are not life-threatening – it's not really a polar bear!

## Emotional eating

When you are in the fight-flight-freeze mode of the primitive brain, your body needs to concentrate on survival, pure and simple. All other non-essential bodily functions can take a bit of a back seat. And one of these is your digestion.

If you were to consider fighting the polar bear or fleeing from it, you would need plenty of energy. The quickest way to get energy would be to grab some sugar, something that gives you an immediate rush. So, your primitive mind commands you eat, and possibly overeat, immediately. And would grab the source of food that gives you the quickest hit of energy: sugar or simple carbs. You can feel out of control with eating as it is the message being received from the primitive brain, a quick survival response. You are eating for your emotions rather than a physical hunger.

Afterwards you may well feel awful and feelings of guilt or shame can consume you. At this point you may have regained intelligent brain control, so begin to look at the situation more objectively and rationally.

When we eat emotionally and mindlessly, we have been consumed by the primitive brain.

If you're in fight-flight-freeze mode your body needs sugar to take action. You want immediate energy. Let's polish off a packet of chocolate biscuits then! And you do this almost without thinking because that primitive emotion drives you to gorge on certain foods.

I often explain to clients that once the stress bucket is empty then they will become more mindful of what and how they eat. Once you do this, you begin to realise that you should be eating for your physical hunger, rather than any sort of emotional void. In simple terms, make sure you eat for your tummy, when you're truly hungry, not for your head.

## Digestive issues

If you were being chased by a polar bear, forget about digesting; you need to run, so digestion can stop altogether. Your primary response is for survival pure and simple. You feel your metabolism is sluggish and slow. It's important to remember here that the opposite of fight or flight is *rest and digest* – you can only digest efficiently when you are calm and relaxed. That's when the digestive juices flow well.

Alternatively, your gut could react in this way: if you needed to escape from the polar bear, it would be good to make yourself lighter so that you could run faster, right? So maybe you'd – how do I put this politely? – 'evacuate your bowel.'

Do you recognise any of these symptoms?

The mind is brilliant at not only recognising stress but sending a message to the rest of the body to take action. In the main, the brain is directly connected to the gut by a huge nerve called the vagus nerve. The brain and the gut are strongly related in this way and communicate with each other easily. This is why more and more often the gut is being referred to by scientists as the *second brain*. I often wonder if this is where the phrases 'your gut feeling' or 'trust your gut' come from.

If you are in a chronic state of stress then it's highly likely you will have some digestive issues and you'll feel that your metabolism is not as efficient as it should be.

For this reason, people who are highly stressed find it very difficult to lose and manage their weight.

It's important to remember here that if the brain can communicate with the body through the vagus nerve then the body can also communicate with the brain. Learning to stimulate healthy function of the vagus nerve by doing things like breathing exercises, can actually send a signal back up to the brain that all is well, there are no polar bears here to panic about.

If you saw a polar bear, naturally your breath would become short and sharp. They would be very rapid breaths from your chest, even leading to hyperventilation.

However, if you consciously take some time to slow your breathing, and breathe a little deeper from deep down in your belly, that will send calming signals upwards via the vagus nerve to your brain.

Here are some simple breathing exercises that can help you do this:

◇ 4-7 breathing. Inhale for the count of four and exhale for the count of seven. As long as your exhale is longer than your inhale then you are sending the right relaxation signals to the brain. For example, you could use 3-6 or 5-9, it's totally up to you.

◇ Focus on your normal breathing but ensure that you breathe from your belly. You can do this by placing one hand on your chest and one on your belly. You should notice the hand on your belly will rise and fall whereas the one on your chest stays relatively still or has minimum movement.

◇ Equal breathing. Focus on your breathing by inhaling through your nose and exhaling through your mouth for equal counts. Usually, a count of 4 for each inhale and exhale is quite nice. This is sometimes known as square, or box, breathing because you can imagine that each inhale and each exhale is one side of a square.

◇ Exhale through your mouth and relax into a pause, then slowly inhale through your nostrils and exhale once again to a pause, for the same count both ways. This method is known as pause breathing and is often used at the beginning of meditation practices.

Now that we can appreciate the evolutionary survival response of the primitive brain, it begs the question: what makes us go into the primitive brain now? If we don't live like cavepeople anymore, why do we still revert to it? In fact, you may even be thinking something like *can't I just switch off my primitive brain – cut it out or something!*

Well, it still has a very useful function. If you stepped out into the road without thinking and a bus beeped at you, you'd jump back! That's your primitive brain at work. The bus driver needs to hit the emergency brake – that's the bus driver's primitive brain at work.

The fire alarm goes off – your primitive brain will make you take action

The good old 'caveman response' still serves us – but we can't let it us consume us. It is ready to hijack us at any point, but we need to remain objective and rational if we want better results. We need to engage our intelligent brain and use that vast resource to help us to live our lives in a calm and relaxed way. This doesn't mean that we deny our problems. It means we can face problems more construct-ively.

**It's not the actual events and things that happen in our lives that cause us to get wrapped up in the primitive brain.**

Everyone has stress in their lives and everyone's had something that has raised their stress levels to an extent they could not have imagined. These are the events of life and the natural order of what makes the world go round too. There's no one on this earth that has never experi-enced a bereavement, financial pressures, family conflict or work stress. You and everyone you know has experienced some stress – no one's lived a charmed life.

So, if it's not the actual events, then what is it?

Well, I believe it's our thought process behind those events. Namely our **negative** thoughts. Negative thinking draws us toward the negative part of our brain and if we're not careful it consumes us.

We can think negatively in two main ways.

We can think negatively about the past, our regrets in life, all those times we failed at something, when relationships failed us, when we didn't get that job we wanted, when things went wrong.

We can also think negatively about the future. We begin to forecast what *will* go wrong. You'll begin to think that you'll never have that car you want; you'll never have the relationship you desire nor the career. Nothing will ever work out right for you.

Now these are quite major thoughts about the big things in life. But it's really important to remember here that this negative forecasting of the future can also apply to those everyday little things in life. In fact, I think that sometimes these are more consuming overall.

You're worried about tomorrow's meeting, how on earth you're going to manage this week's workload, how will you get your coursework in on time. Even something enjoyable like a party – you think you'll hate it and you're not looking forward to it.

Now it's important to remember here that your mind doesn't know the difference between imagination and reality; the imagination can be very powerful indeed. Have you ever watched a horror film? You know that it's only fiction, it's on TV, but your heart is racing and you think Hannibal Lecter is going to jump out at you from behind your sofa! That's how powerful your imagination is, it can make imagined things appear real.

And when we apply this to our thoughts about our life it can be detrimental to our mental wellbeing.

Let's use an example:

Imagine you've got a meeting to go to tomorrow. And you negatively forecast that meeting today. You go over that meeting fifty times in your imagination, negatively, with all the things that will go wrong.

*Why oh why do I have to attend these things? It will be such a waste of time. We won't get an answer to the questions that need asking. Roger is always awful and Karen doesn't stop talking, it'll be a disaster.*

But tomorrow comes along, you attend the meeting and, to your pleasant surprise, it goes quite well. It's been quite productive; Roger seems on top form and Karen was busy at another meeting so couldn't attend anyway. It really didn't turn out quite as bad as you had imagined it.

But, because your mind doesn't know the difference between imagination and reality, your mind now believes that you've been to fifty-one meetings in the last two days and fifty of those have gone badly. It basically can't tell the difference.

Your overall experience therefore is meetings are bad, meetings are bad, meetings are bad – you will rarely remember the one time it was fine.

This also applies to thoughts of the past. If you had a traumatic event happen to you in the past, it's very difficult not to relive it. After all, that's how the mind works, it gets drawn toward the negative. But, like I said, the mind doesn't know the difference between imagination and reality, so if you keep going over that event then it's not only happened once, your mind perceives it to have happened lots of times.

**

### *Paul's story*

Paul was a very successful professional who came to see me as he was consumed with anxiety about, in his words, 'everything'. His sleep was severely affected and although he was in a very loving relationship, he couldn't find the joy in it. In fact, he felt almost guilty that he wasn't able to reciprocate the love and care shown to him by his partner. He was intrigued by my approach as he had a colleague who had come to see me for generalised anxiety and had noticed a huge difference in them quite quickly. His colleague had recommended he come to see me, knowing that Paul was struggling with a lot of issues and was sure that I could help.

At our initial consultation Paul mentioned in passing that he had had a pretty horrific car accident a few years ago. All was fine now but it had left him with thoughts of how his body may be weaker after the trauma and this prevented him from playing rugby which he used to play a lot.

He explained that his thoughts would often take him back to the day of the accident and what had actually happened; he often relived it and although he realised it was not his fault, and no one else was hurt, he still could not get the images out of his mind.

As I explained how the mind works and that it doesn't know the difference between imagination and reality, he slowly looked up at me with tears in eyes and said, 'Gin, so I've not just had that accident once, have I? I've had it about a thousand times now because I keep going over it in my mind.'

It was a powerful realisation for Paul and when I went on to explain that solution-focused work means that I would NOT ask him to go over the accident, or his thoughts and feelings around it, his relief was palpable. He had actually put off coming to see me because of this fear.

Why would I put Paul through that trauma all over again? He had relived it many times over and over again in his mind, he'd unpicked it and examined it. But he didn't feel any better because of it. He needed a different approach. And this didn't mean that we denied the problem, not at all. I wanted him to accept that it had happened, but more importantly, I wanted him to remember that he had survived that accident, and to move on from it. He wanted to feel better and that could only happen if I could help him focus on solutions, help him visualise what he wanted from life right now and where this would take him going forward.

Within a few sessions he was sleeping better and focusing on a more positive future. His relationship improved immensely as we continued with sessions, he was more productive at work and feeling so much happier. He found he really didn't think about his accident any more and even if he did, it was with a very objective and rational view. He completely adored the solution-focused approach and towards the end of sessions wondered why on earth he hadn't been focusing on solutions before, it seemed so obvious now!

\*\*

As you can see from Paul's story, negative thoughts really do have a huge impact on how we feel and consequently behave. And we all have negative thoughts. It's purely that we should try to limit them.

All those negative thoughts about the past and the future, real and imagined, they build up, collect and accumulate in your stress bucket (Yippee – at last, Gin, you've mentioned the stress bucket – I've been waiting ages for this!).

The stress bucket is a metaphor for a part of the brain called the hippocampus, but I'm going to call it a stress bucket for now.

Now I'll let you into a little secret, shhhh don't tell anyone.

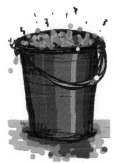

There is a process to empty this bucket!

And you already do it – admittedly you may not be doing it properly now, but you did it a lot as a child – you were never taught how to do it, it came naturally.

In fact, you were born knowing how to do this.

What is it?

Well, it's your sleep.

That's right, sleep empties the stress bucket.

In fact, it's in a specific part of your sleep that this bucket empties, it's a part of your sleep called REM sleep (Rapid Eye Movement).

I bet that once I explain how this works, you'll realise you knew this all along!

## Sleep. It's Free Therapy

To make it easier to understand how sleep empties the stress bucket let's use another example: Let's say someone says something really negative to you one morning. It's so bad that you can't stop thinking about it so you go over it in your thoughts twenty times before you've even had lunch.

It's definitely been stored in your stress bucket. You're really holding onto it.

You carry on with your day as best you can but it seems to keep cropping up in your thoughts through the afternoon. It's now really piling into your stress bucket – it's gone into the bucket about forty times now.

Once you get home, you tell your partner about that awful thing someone said and they say 'oh just forget about it now, will you?' but you can't!

You keep on thinking about it – it's well and truly stuffed into that stress bucket.

When you go to sleep, you go over that event again in your mind's eye, and you're going over it in your REM sleep. You can go over that event realistically or metaphorically, and that's what dreaming is.

When you do this what you're actually doing is removing that thought from the stress bucket and shifting it into the intelligent brain. You're turning that memory from an emotional memory to a very objective one.

It's as if you're taking the emotional sting out of it.

What this means is that when you wake up in the morning you might have forgotten that it happened altogether, but even if you don't, you'll at least have that feeling of *oh, I can't be bothered, that person is not worth me thinking about. Why do I let these kinds of silly people bother me?* and you'll feel you can get on with your day.

This is where those sayings come from: 'things will seem better in the morning', and often if you're worried about something, I'm sure someone's told you to 'sleep on it'.

Think about it – I'm sure there are some stresses that happened yesterday, or even last week, that you've forgotten about. You don't remember that traffic jam you were stuck in, do you? Or when you were running late for that appointment? No, you've processed it out of your stress bucket.

In an ideal world it would lovely to wake up every morning with an immaculately empty stress bucket, so that you can begin your day in the intelligent, objective part of your brain, feeling motivated, positive and raring to go.

What, you don't feel like that? I guess that's why you're reading this book!

Well, there are two reasons that you don't feel as if you've emptied your stress bucket overnight;

Having an empty stress bucket first thing in the morning would be perfectly manageable if there was only one repetitive thought you put into your stress bucket each day. But our minds really love to store a lot more negative thoughts than that.

So, my guess is, you've been piling way too much into your stress bucket. Remember, even imagined negative thoughts can go in there. Have you been going over your regrets again and again? Reliving negative memories? Maybe you're negatively forecasting the future constantly – your imagination is piling all those thoughts into your stress bucket too.

This accumulation of stress in the bucket doesn't happen in one day, it happens over weeks, months, even years sometimes…

Occasionally that bucket can even overflow. That can feel like a real crisis point for some people.

Maybe you need a bigger bucket? Do you need to upgrade to a stress skip?

I know what you're thinking – *well, Gin, how about I do a whole load of REM sleep all in one go – wouldn't that empty the bucket?* If only it was that easy! This leads me to the second reason why you can't empty your stress bucket overnight.

REM sleep should only be about 20% of your sleep at night, you need some deep sleep too. Deep sleep is really physically restorative. It helps revive your muscles and regenerate cells of your body including your vital organs.

If you've got too much in your bucket and you try to do too much REM sleep, your brain is really clever, it recognises this.

Once you hit the 20% mark of REM your brain goes *hang on a minute, this bucket's not empty yet – I want to empty it before morning – what shall I do? More REM please.* Ideally your bucket should be empty within that 20% quota of REM, but as you had piled too much in there, it can sense more work needs to be done.

But it can't do it – your mind wants to switch over to deep sleep. But if the stress bucket's not empty yet it does something else instead; it wakes you up – and it wakes you up at about 3a.m. – wide awake and you can't get back to sleep again. You know the feeling? Waking up at that 'witching hour' when you're wide awake, mind racing, and you have no idea why this happened.

Oh dear, you're now in a vicious circle.

The more you've got in your bucket the more you're encouraged to stay in the primitive brain putting more negative thoughts back into your bucket.

You're now going to undo all the bucket emptying you just did – back to square one!

But not everyone who has an overflowing stress bucket experiences this exactly: There are a small percentage of people that can push through that 20% barrier of REM sleep and stay asleep. Fantastic, you think, who are these people? I want to be one of them.

No, you don't! This isn't good for you either.

By staying asleep and continuing to do REM to empty the bucket sounds great, but it isn't.

REM sleep is draining – it takes up a lot of energy – on top of which you've not had enough deep sleep so, you wake up from eight or nine hours of what you feel is a solid sleep, feeling absolutely exhausted. You will wander around in a bit of a tired stupor, lacking motivation and putting more stress back into your bucket!

**Either way, it's important to remember the excess stress in your bucket is fuel for the primitive brain – it thrives on it!**

So, you'll be driven by the primitive brain now, feeling depressed, anxious and angry, catastrophising, having obsessional thoughts, being vigilant, with a very fixed mindset. You will wake up in the morning with an already half-full stress bucket, so you're already on the back foot to tackle your stress levels. It's so unfair. What a pain!

What you need to do is cut off that fuel supply. You need to empty the bucket of all the excess stress you have accumulated over time. But understanding the basic work-ings of sleep is a huge help in that. I appreciate that you may not feel that you can empty your stress bucket in one good night's sleep, but I will explain how I empty over-flowing stress buckets using solution-focused therapy later. In fact, that is my role now – I empty your stress bucket for you and show you how to keep it empty yourself.

You can make a start right now yourself though, by limiting what goes into the bucket in the first place. I hope what you've read here already will begin to help with that. Now you understand the workings of the brain, observe your thoughts a bit. Notice what part of the brain they are coming from. Are they rational, objective thoughts or primitive, emotional thoughts that come from a sort of survival response? Notice if you're having repetitive, negative thoughts – remember they're no use to you at all. Your mind thinks it's really happening over and over again.

Now don't beat yourself up over how you think. The mind is a fascinating thing, it likes to wander, it likes to take you down random paths. But it's very important to remember that you control your thoughts, they don't control you. They can *feel* like they control you – when you've felt angry and lashed out, when you're feeling sad and want to curl up and cry. But you can control them – you look at photos of your last holiday and it makes you smile. You play with the kids and you can't stop laughing. You can take action to control how you feel.

When you come from the primitive brain it can feel like your thoughts control you – it's your brain trying to look after you and hijacking you into survival mode. But when you come from the intelligent part of your brain you can be more objective and rational. It's in the intelligent brain that you feel you are in control of your thoughts and feelings.

But you'll know when you're managing your stress bucket when you sleep better. Like most things in life, it's about quality over quantity, and it's no different for sleep. You need to ensure that you are getting the right proportions of REM and deep sleep.

Sleep is your new therapy, it's free and you can do it now – well not right now or you won't finish my book, but tonight.

So, you can see that I place a lot of emphasis on sleep. Here are the tips I give most often to help improve sleep immediately:

◇ Monitor your caffeine intake, caffeine has a huge effect on the quality of your sleep.

◇ Try to go to bed at a regular time – get the mind and body used to the routine of going to sleep.

◇ Thirty minutes before bedtime (ideally up to an hour) switch off all digital media. By all means, read, listen to music, relax, but switch off the phone, laptop etc.

◇ Do not take your phone to bed with you – you will remain vigilant. Try to keep the phone out of the bedroom.

◇ Do not watch TV, play video games, or eat in bed. Make the bedroom a place for relaxation and rest.

◇ Make sure your bedroom is cool. It's much easier to fall asleep in a cooler room, you don't want to be hot.

◇ Do not have a heavy meal before bedtime. It's very difficult to sleep on a full stomach.

◇ Same with alcohol. It may feel like it helps you sleep but it is not a sleep aid. You should be able to fall asleep naturally without assistance.

◇ It's nice to have peace but do not expect complete silence. In fact, sometimes complete silence can be disconcerting, remember there will be normal natural sounds but you should not be so vigilant that every tiny sound disturbs you.

Let's face it, deep down you know all of these, and you've probably heard them being recommended all the time. But now that you know *WHY* you need to sleep you should hopefully find yourself doing them.

So, sleep is one important factor in limiting what goes into your stress bucket and I advise that you think carefully about your sleep schedule. I strongly believe that the current mental health epidemic could be vastly reduced by ensuring we value our sleep a lot more.

Unfortunately, things like social media, 24-hour news, video games and a general attitude that being busy is good for you means we are not valuing sleep as much as we should. And yet, doctors are prescribing more and more sleeping pills. Shelves in pharmacies and health food stores are dedicated to sleep aid products. We need to break this cycle.

I often feel stress has got a bit of a bad rap lately. We all think that stress is lots of terrible, unwanted feelings. But it's really important to remember that not all stress is bad for you.

Stress is what happens in your brain and body when you pay attention to something you care about, and that something is at risk now. Even when you cannot do something about it, that is often regarded as stress.

We all need some stress to drive us, to motivate us. People assume that the stress bucket needs to be empty all of the time but that's not real life. Newly graduated university students have this issue a lot. After studying hard for many years, they feel that now they should land the perfect job, meet the perfect partner and live happily ever after. No other stress should come their way because, understandably, they've had enough by that point. But I have to very gently explain life's just not like that. Life will challenge and test us and not everything is within our control. It's important to remember, as I have said before, that maintaining good mental health is not about the actual events that occur but the thought process that goes on around them.

A lot of stressful things can be meaningful – striving to be the best parent you can be, the best at your job, wanting to pass exams or delivering the best presentation you can. Only because you want to do well do you feel that stress, it shows you care about something. It can actually give us some energy and drive.

Some stressful things are out of our control, things you would not choose for yourself, such as illness or bereavements, but even then, you should look at those situations and see if you can harness that stress to meet it, rather than letting it overwhelm you. Can you rise to the challenge? Do you choose to learn from this experience or give in to it?

Your ability to learn from stress is what differentiates your level of resilience from mental illness. The more you do this strengthens the habit of limiting what goes into your stress bucket. Every moment of stress provides you with this opportunity if you choose to take it. Your brain is *always* ready to learn.

I put a bit of stress in my stress bucket every day – it's only natural. But I know that it is a limited amount, well within the amount that my REM sleep will be able to empty for me overnight.

This limited amount of stress in our stress bucket is known as challenge stress – just enough to challenge and drive us. This is the type of stress that helps us meet deadlines, be punctual and work towards goals. It's really good for us. It enables us to learn, grow and adapt.

But once you start piling too much into the bucket, too much for 20% REM sleep to cope with, then that type of stress feels more aggressive and is therefore called threat stress. This type of stress fuels the primitive brain, because it's too much for your REM at night to cope with. You wake up in the morning with this residual stress left over, therefore even challenge stress feels menacing.

Your job is to make sure you can recognise the difference between what is a threat and what is a challenge. Regularly facing some challenge stress builds resilience and ensures a more long-term, healthy approach to dealing with life's issues. It's really important that you can embrace the mindset that surrounds positive types of stress, knowing that your brain can defend itself against it, learn from it and become stronger from it too.

Stress is actually trying to help us engage with life, this is an innate response within all of us.

# The 3 P's

N ow you are beginning to understand brain function, and the importance of sleep, it's time to look at other active processes you can use to manage your thoughts and feelings effectively to help you empty your stress bucket.

### 'I'll do that when I feel better.'

How many times have you said this to yourself? – When I feel better, I'll get back to normal, I'll pick up that hobby, I'll do that thing I like.

What are you waiting for?

When will you feel better?

Feeling better doesn't happen by magic! You have to take some positive action to feel better. You should be saying I will do that thing and that will make me feel better...which means I can do more of that thing and other stuff I enjoy too. It's a continuous cycle.

The caveman knew this! When the caveman lived in their tribe properly, did their hunting and gathering, socialised and rested well, they felt really good. They were happy and motivated.

In fact, they didn't know this at the time, but what they got was a biological reward. This biological reward was a boost of the happy hormone, serotonin. Yippee, they felt great!

Try to think about times when you've had a 'natural high'. It's been times when you've been happy, you've had good feelings flowing inside you. Yes, it may be due to a significant event in your life but remember the cycle…you're in control. The people I know with great mental health value all the small things in their life that brings them small bursts of joy and excitement. They can find the joy in the smallest of things. In fact, they deliberately build those things into their daily routine. You can make things happen to create that boost of serotonin in yourself.

Luckily, we don't have to do exactly what the caveman did and go out and club a woolly mammoth over the head to feed our tribe, nor do we need have huge significant events all the time. In fact, if you had significant events all the time, they wouldn't be significant, would they?

But you do need to take those caveman principles and apply them to modern times.

## You need to do the three P's

No, that's not garden peas – the letter P! The letter P stands for Positive.

### 1) Positive Activity

Find an activity that is positive for you. Exercise is the one that comes to mind but if that has a negative connotation, reframe it as movement. Walking or swimming for example.

We are not actually evolved or designed to hit the gym. We are, however, designed to move. We hunted, gathered and foraged before we sat down to eat. These days we merely need to press a few buttons on our phone and we can have food delivered to our door within minutes. We're not really earning our food any more.

This *inconsequential movement* that we did through evolution really made a difference. Our lifestyles have changed so much now though that we are much more sedentary than ever, often at desks for long periods of time. We therefore overcompensate this by hitting the gym hard. We need to find more balance.

If you enjoy the gym and running marathons then all well and good, but make sure you are not stressed out when you do it – your mind will perceive it as if you are literally running away from the polar bear.

But if you can't bear the thought of a gym then can you reframe your exercise into the word **movement** instead – just move more. Walking, dancing, running around after the kids or rushing about with the vacuum cleaner. All movement counts.

Positive activities also include your hobbies as well. Your positive activity may be gardening or knitting. How about a jigsaw puzzle even? Remember it's got to be positive for you.

One of my friends loves running. She's always telling me about the fantastic benefits of it, how good she feels afterwards, and even during when she hits that 'runner's high!' And that's great for her. She always tries to get me out on a run with her. But I hate running – it's not *my* positive activity. I do love the outdoor bootcamp I attend, I really love yoga, and I can walk for miles…they're my positive activities.

Make a list of *your* positive activities. Make sure you have access to the tools or equipment you need to do them. Many activities don't require anything at all. Knowing that *you* enjoy doing them is enough. I guarantee doing more of your positive activities will get your serotonin flowing.

## 2) Positive Interactions

Human beings are social animals, we like being part of a community or 'tribe'.

Make sure you spend time with people that you feel positive simply being around. There are just those people that are a joy to be with. We all know who they are in our circle. And it doesn't have to be in person.

You know that person you get off the phone from and you feel so happy after talking to them.

That person who always send cards in the post – aren't those people lovely?

They are your positive interactions. Being around these people and interacting with them makes us feel good, and if you feel good, you'll also give off more positive vibes encouraging more people to feel good, thus building your tribe.

We can even include animals in this. I challenge you not to feel positive after playing with a dog or cat. Look after your pets and they will look after you. So, whether you've got a horse or a lizard, nurture that positive interaction.

Stress can actually strengthen relationships; it can give you the energy to turn to someone for help or to focus more on someone you care about instead of navel-gazing. It activates the primitive response of wanting to be part of the tribe.

## Mood hoovers:

Now, there are those people in our lives who can be negative interactions. You feel drained and exhausted after speaking with them.

Unfortunately, we can't always avoid those negative interactions. They can be part of our direct family, living with us. Or colleagues that we must interact with to get the work done. If this is the case, be extra careful. Knowing that this will affect your flow of serotonin, you may need to be more guarded. Imagine a brick wall around you where everything bounces off, or imagine yourself in a bubble. I assure you that once your stress bucket empties it will become easier, as you gain more objectivity and more rational control. Your level of acceptance will also increase dramatically.

Recognise negative interactions for what they are and guard yourself against them. Especially if you are feeling vulnerable. You can always go back to them at a later date if you wish and feel able, but look after yourself first and limit the interaction you have with them. In fact, if you can go back to them with more positivity then you could even influence them to improve *their* mood.

### 3. Positive Thinking

Of the three P's this is the most difficult.

And I don't say 'think positive' easily.

If there is one thing that fills up my stress bucket it's all those 'think positive' memes, GIFs and graphics all over social media – you know the ones – there's a photo of a beautiful woman with amazing hair and skin and in fancy font it says 'think positive' – well, honey, if I looked like you, I'd be thinking positive too! Don't get me started!

It isn't enough to only think positive – we need to take positive action to do that. It's not a switch you can flick at the back of your head to go from negative to positive. Positive actions and positive interactions will help you to think positively. So, concentrate on 1 and 2, and number 3 will come in time.

The chapter 'What's been good?' will help you with this too.

**

### Uncle Lalli's story

I'm very lucky that my family has roots in India and we now use this as our holiday home. It's a place where my dad grew up, but where I can see my living family tree with its branches walking before me. I visit regularly. I remember my dad talking to one of my uncles in India while we were holidaying there one year.

Now this uncle is a hulk of a man – over six foot tall with hands like spades! He was always a cheerful soul and had some great stories to tell. But, with a potted history of bereavement and loss, it seemed as if life had caught up with him at the age of sixty-five and he had begun to give up. He lost motivation and had become very quiet. We had heard from his son and wife that he also attempted to commit suicide recently, they had luckily managed to stop him in time but they were now really fearful that he would attempt it again. Uncle Lalli had slowly and gradually become more and more depressed over the course of a year.

So much so, that he had begun to neglect his farming duties, which involve quite a lot of manual work. He had begun to withdraw himself from his extensive family and had lost his appetite for food as well as life. My dad was trying to encourage him to get back out to his land, attend to his crops, but Uncle Lalli kept talking about his losses of the past. He said he would get back to his land when he felt better.

But when would he feel better? It was awful to see him this way. He needed to do some positive activity to get his serotonin flowing. He needed some positive interactions. He seemed to be in a vicious circle of lacking motivation to do anything, and yet we knew that doing something, especially on his farm, where he would be interacting with his farm labourers and his cattle, would definitely make him feel better. How could he break the cycle?

And so, while he was trying to coax Uncle Lalli out of his dark mood, Dad began doing a bit of weeding in his courtyard. Except, he deliberately did it incorrectly, making mistakes he knew Uncle Lalli would not be able to sit and watch without at least saying something. But in fact, this was enough to get Uncle Lalli out of his chair and begin to show Dad how to do it right. While they were doing this, Dad joked that he had always come to Uncle Lalli for farming advice even when they were teenagers. He complimented Uncle Lalli on his knowledge and experience and went on to ask him some advice on some of the current crops and how the season would affect them. Slowly and gradually, as Uncle Lalli began to work with his hands, and share his farming expertise with Dad, bringing back positive memories of the past, his focus returned to the present, literally to the task in hand. I could almost see the serotonin begin to flow and a small smile appear on his face. It was as if Dad was coaxing him out of his cave.

I didn't even realise Dad was a secret psychotherapist!

Over the next few weeks, Uncle Lalli re-engaged with life, got back to his farm, and when I saw him again the following year, was an even better version of the joyful, jolly Uncle Lalli I had always known. He had found his purpose again.

Never underestimate how being consistent with your small positive activities, having positive interactions, and focusing on positive memories of the past, can maintain your mental health.

**\*\***

Remember, don't just sit and wait to feel better – take positive action, have positive interactions and THEN you'll begin to feel better – you'll get that boost of the happy hormone and feel motivated to do more – thus continuing the cycle in an upward spiral.

These three P's are often underrated and can seem like hard work when your stress bucket is full. The easier option, particularly with all the advancements in medical science, is to take antidepressants or anti-anxiety medication.

And they can prove hugely beneficial. I am not against medication at all. However, these medications do not directly produce serotonin. That is only something you can do yourself by doing your three P's.

Most modern-day antidepressants are SSRI's (selective serotonin reuptake inhibitors). They are designed to slow down the reuptake of serotonin. But if you're not producing any serotonin in the first place, which is what depression is, then there is nothing to 'inhibit'.

Antidepressants are designed to give you a bit of a boost of serotonin over time to give you just enough encouragement to get back into your three P's. Once you're doing your three P's, you will be able to get more serotonin to flow through you, and the positive upward cycle of feeling better and doing more good things continues.

I have no objection to anyone taking medication to improve their mental health, but understand how they work and how they can benefit you. Use them to give yourself the boost you need to empty your stress bucket.

## Addiction

Often, if we cannot find the motivation to create our own serotonin by doing our three P's, we can easily look externally for an easier 'reward' system to give us that boost of happiness we crave. Things like alcohol and food may fill that gap. This can also develop into more serious issues of addiction, and people search for even more dangerous resources like gambling and illegal drugs, craving that chemical hook to make themselves feel better.

But what we currently know about addictions can be misinterpreted.

There was a really interesting series of studies published in 1978 and 1981 called 'Rat Park' by a Canadian psychologist called Bruce K. Alexander and his colleagues at Simon Fraser University in British Columbia, Canada.

They took a study from early in the 20th century and examined it carefully. In this earlier study rats had been given a choice of two water bottles. One bottle was plain water but the other was water laced with heroin. It was consequently proved that the rats became addicted to the drugged water and kept coming back to it for more and more, until they died.

But Bruce and his team felt this experiment was flawed. They noticed that the rats had been put into individual cages, so the only joy they had was to take the drugs, it made them feel good. What would happen if they changed that? *How* could they change that? Well, what the team did was to build Rat Park; a utopia for rats where there were lots of fun activities. They had balls to play with, a lot of open space, tunnels to scabble down, and lots of rat friends to interact and socialise with. All their needs were fulfilled.

They still had the two water bottles, one plain, one laced with heroin. But guess what? In Rat Park the rats hardly ever drank the drugged water, they were more than happy with the plain water. Even if they occasionally drank some of the drugged water, they didn't become addicted to it. They found so much joy in other things they didn't need the drugs, unlike the rats in the original study that were lonely and had no stimulation.

This doesn't only happen in rats.

During the Vietnam war the use of drugs, in particular heroin, was rife. Some statistics show that up to 20% of American troops were using the drug. Let's face it, if you were forced at a young age to go to fight in a war that you didn't believe in, in fear of being killed or having to kill, then maybe heroin would provide a great mental escape from that. The US government was extremely concerned that once the war was over, they would have a returning generation of junkies landing back with them.

But they needn't have worried, it turned out that 95% of returning veterans simply stopped taking drugs as soon as they got home. That didn't make sense – heroin is addictive, right? And this is what I mean when I say our old theories of addiction are wrong.

What became apparent was that when these veterans got back home to their loving families, got back into things they enjoyed and found purpose in their work again, they didn't need to escape from that. It was like they went from individual cages to a human Rat Park.

So, it's really about the environment you are in and what you can create for yourself. As humans we are social beings, we want to bond and connect (positive interactions), we like to be active and do nice things (positive activity) which makes us feel happy and content (positive thinking).

We need to think about addiction differently. It's a symptom of the disconnection we feel all around us. When you are run down by life, isolated, reliving past traumas and hurts, the motivation to do anything at all is absent. You might look for that sense of relief elsewhere instead, maybe endlessly scrolling social media feeds, playing violent video games, gambling or cocaine! These are unhealthy bonds.

So, we must do the three P's in order to create healthier bonds. Don't prioritise material things over connection.

I always try to listen out to what my clients have been doing during their week, if they have been doing plenty of positive activity and having lots of positive interactions. And it's often the small things that are most powerful in helping to maintain a good flow of serotonin. We can't go on holiday every week or go to a party every single day. It's important to remember that we should be trying to fit in small positive actions and interactions into our everyday lives. It should feel a natural part of our routine.

# What's Been Good?

Now that you understand some basics of how the brain works, and how doing your three P's can give you a positive biological boost, let's look at the active talking processes of solution-focused therapy I use during sessions and how that can empty your stress bucket even quicker.

Hopefully, you have gathered by now that the whole idea is to 'step away' from the primitive brain, calming it down, so that you can be more present in your intelligent brain. In the intelligent brain, as well as feeling calm and relaxed, you will feel more in control of your thoughts and feelings, more objective and rational.

So here is a surefire, quick and easy way to do that:

Instead of asking 'how are you?' – change that to 'what's been good?'

Whether you're talking to others or thinking about how you feel yourself, ask THAT question and that question only.

What's been good about your day? What's been good about your week?

Can you see the difference? Can you *feel* the difference?

When you're asked how you are, I bet you'll say fine, even if you don't mean it. Even if you do mean it, you might say something like 'fine, good, but I had this awful stressful situation and then this terrible thing happened and it's raining as well'.

If you focus only on how you're feeling right now, you are on alert for the negatives, you want to ensure that nothing is 'wrong'.

Our mind naturally wants to go to the negative. It's a survival response. Everything needs to get filtered through the primitive brain for survival.

By asking instead 'what's been good?' we are trying to fully engage the intelligent brain, the positive part of our brain, in fact, we are trying to literally think positive.

Now all my sessions begin with that question – 'What's been good about your week?'

I'm not looking for anything major here but I'm looking for some positive things that have happened to you recently.

Here are a few of the favourites I've heard over the years:

*I saw a cute dog and the owner let me pet him.*

*My chickens were sunbathing* (I got sent a photograph by the way – it became my screensaver!)

*I played with my little girl and out of the blue she told me how much she loved me.*

*My boss is on holiday* – I initially wondered why this was good as I assumed that there would be increased workload, but was told that *we hate our boss so the office atmosphere is much improved* – great – it's your good thing, I'll take it!

*I had a beautiful walk in the rain.*

*I finished watching that series on TV – it was great* (I think it was *Line of Duty* – if you've never watched it, it's amazing!)

I was once told *Oh, I forgot to tell you another good thing, Gin, I inherited £10,000* (this was told to me on leaving the session – crazy how the negative mind is so in control when we're stressed. Only when relaxed did they tell me of this huge windfall!)

But it's the little things in life that keep us going. We can't expect large events like inheritances to keep coming in order to lift our mood. We need to begin to feel more grateful for the little things in life

Now this isn't supposed to be a memory game. Even while you are *trying* to think of good things you are exercising the intelligent brain. But if you'd like to start writing them down that's good too. If you wrote down two things that were good every day, in a week you'd have fourteen things, in a month you'd have sixty things, in three months...I could go on but you catch my drift!

However, write down as many as you can. Ask yourself what else? What else? What else has been good? This way you are strengthening the nerve connections in the intelligent brain and the primitive brain is getting bored.

I continually ask my clients, what else has been good…and tell me another thing that has been good about your week. We can carry on for 10–15 minutes, or longer once the stress bucket is empty. And when they think I've stopped asking and will move on to the next part of our session, I always ask for 'just one more good thing about your week'.

The primitive caveman brain thinks *What? You're not asking me anything negative – hey, I've got something to say*. But no, what's been **good** about your week/your day is the only thing you want to think about for a moment, this engages the intelligent, rational and positive part of your brain. And by continually asking 'what else?' the primitive brain begins to get bored and calms down.

If you keep a record of these things over time, and in particular when you feel low or anxious, you can look back on your notes and remember those things that happened or that you were thankful for and you will shift your mood.

Remember your mind doesn't know the difference between imagination and reality, so you're experiencing that good time again. I bet there will be things on that list that you had forgotten about, maybe quite significant things. The brain wants to draw you to the negative, it takes conscious effort to go to the positive. So be patient with yourself and don't rush.

But like any muscle in the body – repetition will strengthen it.

Recently this sort of thing has been called gratitude journaling. When words like that are thrown about, I tend to find that sometimes people's eyes glaze over, as if it's some New Age fad. But when I explain *why* you should do this, I find many of my clients get on board with it and actually begin to keep a list of all their good things. Once you understand the logical reason why, you're more likely to agree to do it.

This is also a good game to play with family and friends. Try it around the dinner table.

Maybe you could try to respond positively when someone asks you how you are. Then ask *them* what's been good. Initially they won't hear you, they'll go straight to the negative, but correct them: 'hang on a minute – I asked you what's been good, not what's been bad.'

It takes some practice and initially it can feel very unnatural but I guarantee you, this stuff works. After only a few tries you'll get the hang of it.

Now by asking only about the good things of your week I don't for one minute think that you have not had any stress or strain. Life's not like that. Of course, there has been stress this week. But let's not continue to put it into our stress bucket.

It's just that we don't want to give it too much thought, we don't want to activate the primitive brain. And it doesn't mean that all your problems will disappear by doing this exercise, but by activating the intelligent brain you can use your positive, objective and rational resources to tackle your problems and issues, rather than being in a primitive, emotional state. It's very important that each and every solution-focused session begins in the intelligent brain, and this is the easiest way to get there.

To keep this up constantly though is very difficult, nigh on impossible. Remember, you have to filter things naturally through the negative part of your brain, it's simply a survival response. But by taking some time out of your day or week to sit with the thought of what's been good about your week, will help you begin to think positively.

So, I challenge you to change your words to *what's been good?* Ask it more often, make a game of it with the family – the mood will be so much lighter.

And when people ask you how you are – reply with something that has been good for you, something positive. You'll be surprised at the response you feel and I'm sure you'll illicit a more positive response from others as well.

Go on – try it!

At the end of this book, I have included a six-week positivity journal to help with this.

# Solution-Focused Therapy

So now you've got the basics, how do I train people's brains? What is the actual process I use and how can you use this to empty your own stress bucket?

Well, having this knowledge of how your brain works is a start.

But here are some of the other tools I use to help people empty their stress buckets quickly. These can all be easily used on yourself too, and it's a great way to begin to train your brain into a more solution-focused way of thinking. Remember the principle is to cut off the fuel supply to the primitive brain by emptying the stress bucket, so you will shift towards the intelligent brain where you will be more objective, rational and in control of your thoughts and feelings.

## Scaling

There's something about numbers and scales that appeals to me – it makes things more practical, and visualising things in numeric form can make them clearer.

I use something called a happiness scale quite a lot. I like to think of this scale as a gauge, I can gauge my feelings, and I can compare them too. This is a scale from 10–0.

I'm using the word **happiness** here quite loosely. It's not about being all smiley and jovial. It's really about whatever happiness means to you. Maybe happiness to you means feeling in control, feeling more capable, that you're managing and feel mentally strong. Maybe happiness is more about feeling confident and assertive, or maybe it's more about being calm and laid-back. It's the goal that you want to reach, a place you will feel absolutely fulfilled and content.

On the happiness scale number 10 is the epitome of your definition of happiness – the best you could be. And 0 is the other end of the scale, where everything is a complete disaster.

What number would you say you are on that scale right now? Not what number you'd like to be but the number you feel right now. Hold onto that number and we will come back to it in a moment.

It's important now to also create a bit of context around this scale so let's look at the other numbers on it.

So, looking at that scale, in your lifetime, what's lowest number you've ever been and what's the highest? When I ask clients this it gives me some context, but what it should do for you is show you that you have had good times in your life. You've had some real highs. It will also naturally let you know and appreciate there have been low times too but that you survived them and got through.

Now for the highest number, hopefully, you've said 10 but often people will say 8 or 9, because they want something more to work towards and that's fine.

Whatever your highest number is on that scale, I'd like you to think about the actual times when you've been that number. Think back to those wonderful times and how you were feeling, how elated you were, your sense of confidence and achievement.

At this point maybe you'd like to look up some photos of those times, or certificates, or any notes you have around those events. This will all help to bring back those positive memories.

Maybe it was some good holidays or social occasions. Or perhaps when you achieved a goal in further education, or received an award, maybe it was when you first met your partner or had your children. Take a few moments to think about those high points on the scale.

Remember we are keeping it solution focused so you'll notice I asked you to think about the lowest number but not the details of it. That's because I don't want you to dwell on it. We can appreciate you've had low times but we don't need to go over them. Just take time thinking of the good things only.

Now comes the entertaining bit. Let's go back to the number that you feel you are right now this very minute. We're going to play a little game with that number, and have some fun with it. We're about to nudge your mind into a positive direction and create some real brain change. Here we go!

I'd like you to imagine that you carry on with the rest of your day as normal but tomorrow, or maybe one day later on this week, you wake up in the morning and you are magically one step up that scale, you're one step closer to 10.

So, if you said you were a 3 imagine you woke up and you were a 4.

If you think you're a 7 now imagine you woke up an 8.

Whatever number you are I want you to only add 1 to it.

I'm not going to make you jump to 10 and there's reason for that;

There is too much room for error.

Let's say you were feeling a 3 and I asked you to imagine 10 – well, that's just too far to jump – how on earth, overnight or in a few days, would that happen, it's impossible. Your primitive brain will look at all the things that could go wrong – it won't let it happen, it's too far-fetched.

And even if you thought you were 8 it's still quite a leap to 10. 10 is perfection, you know intelligently it's going to take nothing short of an overnight miracle to make that happen and we don't want to alert the primitive brain – so +1 is fine for now, wherever you are on the scale. Small steps only.

We already got the primitive brain a bit bored by asking about all the good things about your week. We want to continue to keep it relaxed and calm, so we don't need to alert it to any sense of danger now.

Now if you were to wake up at that new number on the scale what would be different?

What would feel different? What would have changed?

It's important to remember here that it's not about what you would do to make you feel that new number. Imagine magic has occurred and you actually ARE that number. Take it from there. You will already know what kind of things make you feel better, you are referring to old patterns of behaviour. You're referring to old templates in your brain, that may have been useful at one point in time. This is a useful thing to do but it does not really create new change in the brain. And if you know these things work then why aren't you doing them already? It's because your primitive brain won't let you right now. If you want to create a shift in your way of thinking, you need to be quite careful about this.

Solution-focused work relies on the premise that you can get creative and think of new things. Remember it's only an idea, we're using your imagination, so treat it like a bit of a game if that helps. It's almost as if we want your imagination to get a bit more excited than normal.

Once you've done this, you now need to get a bit more specific because the brain loves details.

I'd like you to think of a small but definite thing that you would be doing that would show you that you feel that way.

What in particular would you do differently if you felt that way? And what would be good about that?

This need only be a small act, maybe something you do anyway but you want to imagine doing it a little better, as if you were that +1 step up on the scale. What we're trying to create is what we call a 'doing picture', remember it's not enough to think positive we need to turn that thought into action. And we're just using our imagination at this stage.

The specificity of this act must be noted quite clearly. Where would you be doing this? What time would it be? Would anyone else be there?

Try to do that now.

Get specific – build a detailed 'doing picture'.

Once you have a clear, detailed 'doing picture' I want you to look at it, really visualise it and ask yourself if it fills you with a sense of being pleased with yourself. Is that a positive, quite interesting picture for you? If not, you may need to go back and start again.

For example:

Let's say you feel a 3 right now, and you wake up tomorrow and you're magically a 4, a tiny step up. By waking up feeling a 4 you might say that you feel a little more rested with a bit more energy than the day before.

Now if you had a bit more energy what would you be doing? An example would be that you would get out of bed without hitting the snooze button and jump straight in the shower to get ready. Remember we're using your imagination, think of what you would do if you had a bit more energy.

What time would you jump in the shower? What room of your house is that (I know it's the bathroom but I need you to really visualise *your* actual bathroom in your own mind)?

Would you be pleased if that happened? Is that a good feeling? – to jump out of bed without hitting snooze with lots of energy and jump straight into the shower – great stuff! What a brilliant 'doing picture'.

Maybe a typical example of one of my sessions with a client called Sam will help clarify that. In this example I have shown a slight variation in that I ask Sam what particular thing would ensure that the action she would take tomorrow would happen. This works equally as affectively as thinking of an event happening in the future, and I use this variation more in cases of depression as it is a little easier for the mind:

Me: On your happiness scale, if number 10 is where you want to be, and 0 is the other end of that scale, what number would you say you are on that scale right now?

Sam: I'm a 5.

Me: Great, right in the middle there (note I will always give you positive feedback at each step – your mind needs to hear that you are doing well so that it is encouraged to keep going. Even if you said you felt number 1 – I'd still say that was good – better than 0!).

Now use your lovely imagination, let's say you go to bed tonight and overnight I wave a magic wand and you wake up tomorrow morning and you're a 6 on that scale. What would be different?

Sam: I would wake up, ready for the day, feeling very motivated and organised.

Me: Fabulous. How would you know you're feeling motivated and organised?

Sam: Well, my clothes for the day will be laid out ready so that I can jump in the shower and get ready quickly.

Me: Sounds good! What particular thing would ensure that that happened?

Sam: I guess I will have laid out my clothes for the day the night before, that would be the best thing, tonight then, I'll lay my clothes out ready tonight.

Me: (I want the details) Lovely, and when exactly will you do that, what time will it be?

Sam: I'll do that tonight before I got to bed at about 9.30p.m.

Me: And *where* will you be doing that?

Sam: I'd be doing that in my bedroom and laying them out on the chair in the corner of my room.

Me: (I will summarise) So let's imagine that you've woken up tomorrow and you're feeling a 6 on the scale, you know you're a 6 because you feel ready for the day, motivated and organised. And one thing that makes you feel organised is seeing that your clothes are out and ready for the day ahead. And your clothes are ready because tonight at 9.30p.m. you got them ready by being in your bedroom and laying them out on the chair in the corner. So, if you imagine yourself tonight at 9.30p.m., in your bedroom, getting your clothes ready and laying them out on the corner chair, how does that make you feel? Would you be pleased?

Sam: Oh yes, I'd be really pleased, in fact, I'd be quite proud of myself.

Me: Well done, Sam. A brilliant 'doing picture'.

Now this may seem like a small act but remember what we're doing. We are nudging the mind into the right direction, the positive direction, without alerting the primitive brain. This small act, hopefully, makes you feel motivated, organised and even proud. If we can elicit these positive feelings now it will make the next step of the process so much more effective.

Now I am not going to hold Sam to this decision, I'm not going to make sure she did it when I see her next week. It's just an idea, a thought, something that makes Sam feel good. The mind appreciates that and will work with it now, to come up with other solutions that make her feel motivated, organised and proud. We need to let the mind get a bit creative with this idea but it is initiated by the feelings it creates not the actions themselves. And anyway, the mind doesn't know the difference between imagination and reality so it's as if she's already done it!

It's not necessary to go away and actually do that thing. More often than not you may find that you do but it's not necessarily the point of this exercise. Let your imagination do all the work at this point.

Getting this picture right, getting a positive feeling from it is really important. Make sure it's something realistic and practical – almost as if the primitive brain will be bored by it. In our example above, Sam's primitive brain would maybe react with: *What Sam? That's it – you'll get your clothes ready for tomorrow – well, that is so mundane that nothing could go wrong there –* it's quite a simple act.

However, we do want to nudge the mind in the right direction, so it has to give some sort of positive feeling, not only a nice feeling but a quite excited and motivated sort of feeling.

In the above example, Sam lacked so much motivation and was not really planning her days very well at all. Even the thought of doing this, which she knew deep down would be really helpful, made her feel happy.

You've got to try and hit that sweet spot where your 'doing picture' creates a joyful feeling within you.

Now this scale is quite arbitrary and for sure the definition of the extent of the scale can vary quite a bit. What number 10 will be on your scale in six months' time will be very different to what it is now. But that's because once you hit the number 10, you'll move your own goal posts, and that's what keeps you moving forward. So, every time you do this exercise do not compare yourself to what you were last time, or predict too far ahead where on the scale you feel you need to be. Treat it as a separate exercise each time you do it.

Now if your 'doing picture' does not meet those criteria simply go back and start again – make sure you get that nudge just right.

It's quite tricky to create a clear 'doing picture' initially, but you really can't make a mistake here so don't worry if you find this difficult to begin with, you'll get there. Do the best you can. It takes a bit of practise. Go with the best 'doing picture' you can think of.

## Unconscious Bias

Unconscious bias is the brain's way of making a quick judgement without engaging rational thought processes.

It's really important you get your language right to continue to think positively, so that you're not unknowingly creating bias towards a certain way of thinking. You need to engage that rationale and objectivity of the intelligent brain. And to do this you need to understand how your brain translates language.

For example, right now I'm going to ask you not to think about a green bus. Don't think about it – no, stop it – don't think about a green bus!

What are you thinking about? A green bus, right? But I asked you NOT to think about a green bus!

The mind does not 'hear' the 'not' in front of it – it only hears 'green bus, green bus, green bus'. So, it's really important to make sure you use the right language.

Think about a red bus – OK, that's more like it! Does that make sense?

When have you really wanted something and you go out and that's all you see?

I love shoes – trainers in particular (I'm all about the comfort me!) So, when I see a nice pair online or in a magazine, I think *ooh, I'd love them*. I do a bit more research online finding out about cost, looking at more pictures of them, and finding out where they're available.

The next day, on the way to get my groceries, I see two people wearing those trainers and an advert at the bus stop for them. I come home and the shop they're available in has an advert on the TV.

That didn't happen by chance. Those people would have worn their trainers anyway, the advert has been at the bus stop for a week already, and I happened to turn on the TV at the right time – BUT my subconscious was now alerting me – oh, Gin, there's those trainers you were thinking about, oh there they are again, and again!

It's like making a shopping list – you make a list of what you want – not what you don't want!

Your mind is drawn to what you think of.

It's no good to keep saying to yourself 'I DON'T want to feel anxious' or 'I DON'T want to feel depressed' – because now your mind is directed towards anxiety and depression.

In fact, your subconscious mind will look for ways to prove that to you, and that's unconscious bias. You may even feel the physical symptoms that prove to you that you're feeling anxious.

You will cry a lot easier at the smallest things because you've told yourself you feel sad. You can feel the butter-flies in your stomach because of your nervousness.

What you should think about is what you want to feel instead. And this is really important when you are creating your 'doing picture'. You may think that waking up tomor-row, feeling one step higher on your happiness scale, would mean that you weren't feeling so tired. Using the principle I just explained, you're still thinking about tiredness. So, if that is how you initially phrase the answer, don't panic, ask yourself – well, what would I be feeling instead?

You would have more energy. This is much more positive and solution-focused language.

Calm, happy, relaxed maybe. More confident, or motivated.

Now this takes some effort and practice.

But you don't go to the gym once and expect amazing muscles, do you?

When you were a child learning to walk, you didn't give up the first time you fell over. You didn't think, *oh, this walking lark is not for me; I fell.* You kept on trying and trying – until you can now walk without thinking!

Use this same principle to train your brain – it's no 'secret' or law of attraction. It's the scientific, logical way that your brain works. It takes practice and time, but I have seen people turn their whole way of thinking around simply by remembering this one principle and applying it consistently. Not giving up if they fail occasionally.

Unconscious bias is powerful – don't misjudge it.

## Relaxation and the Default Mode Network

You can use scaling and the doing picture whenever you want to. In solution-focused therapy sessions, in order to create tangible change in the brain we will combine it with deep relaxation. As soon as you have your 'doing picture' and it is framed in the correct language, it's time to relax.

There are many forms of relaxation that you can utilise and just resting and going to sleep is one of them. So, you can do this exercise before you go to bed at night. In fact, to begin with, I'd suggest exactly that.

You can also do things like meditation and mindfulness if you feel confident and able to do so.

And you don't have to sit in the lotus position under a tree and chant with joss sticks surrounding you!

There is a third option.

And it's this option that I encourage the most. I find meditation and mindfulness quite challenging actually. Do you know how hard it is to focus on one thing? Apparently, Buddhist monks go on thirteen-year retreats into the Himalayas to really train their mind to meditate. So, if you've got a spare thirteen years then feel free, but there is an easier way.

The easy third option is to do nothing. Allow your mind to wander and get a bit bored. Just stop, close your eyes and do zilch, zero, nada. The mind has a natural propensity to wander. Let it. This is your mind's way of emptying the stress bucket.

In sessions at this point I do a guided relaxation exercise focusing on the body relaxing and then some visualisations, often around nature, things like trees and lakes. But I expect your mind to wander here. You may begin to think about what you're going to have for dinner, or that meeting you've got to prepare for. It really doesn't matter. It's really important that you can feel relaxed enough to do nothing.

If you really feel that this is a bit too much of doing absolutely nothing, then try going for a walk on your own and don't take your phone with you. That's right, no headphones, nothing, allow your mind to daydream.

The important thing is to make sure it is the same thing – something you can do almost without thinking about it. As if you're on autopilot. So, I would not recommend you do something like drive or watch a documentary, you do need to switch off completely.

Ideally a relaxation recording of some sort should do the trick. There are lots of things you can access online for free these days, so find some relaxing music settle down and chill out.

The reason people find this difficult is that we have never before lived in an age where we have so much information at the tips of our fingers, always something to be doing, reading, or listening to. We rarely do nothing at all, it's like we need to be constantly stimulated. It can also be regarded as lazy to do nothing at all, but your mind needs the down time, it needs the space to empty the stress bucket.

At this juncture, where you have created a detailed, positive 'doing picture' and you are ready to go into relaxation, the mind is very clever – it's working with the idea of something that makes you feel good and, if you can relax completely, it's coming up with more ideas around that – your mind always works on what you direct it towards. And it's working really hard. You're not just switching off; you are, in fact, switching over to another state in which your subconscious can get to work without interference from the conscious parts of your brain for a small amount of time. This is known as the Default Mode Network (DMN).

The DMN is a goal-oriented brain state, that comes up with solutions to problems, gets creative with new ideas and increases motivation. How many times have you sat at your desk worrying about a problem, but you go for a quick walk at lunchtime and when you return to your desk, it seems that the solution jumps out to you? That's the DMN at work.

To activate the DMN you need to relax and almost get bored. It's a subconscious state of mind that you can do automatically. It's very organic and you may already be engaging it without even realising.

When you've driven a long distance and can't remember how you got there, that's the DMN engaged and at work. Or if you've watched a good film or read a good book and can't believe two hours have passed – that's the DMN at work again.

It's not like you are putting your brain into screensaver mode. Not at all. Your brain is very much at work. You're activating a different part of the brain, regions rather than your conscious, intelligent parts. They are your medial pre-frontal cortex, medial parietal cortex and medial temporal lobes. There is still a bit of a mystery in science about what actually goes on in these areas when we allow our mind to wander. What we do know is that a huge amount of electrical activity occurs in these areas when we relax and daydream, allowing our mind to wander.

This is separate from conscious thought. One theory, and the one that I rely on for solution-focused work, is that when the DMN is activated the brain is consolidating experiences and preparing to react to the environment. The DMN is taking all that conscious thought and turning it into something more understandable, organising and planning to come up with new ideas and new ways of thinking. It's also open to learning and absorbing new ideas.

Allow your mind to relax, allow your imagination to wander, it is really very powerful.

That's why I love the solution-focused way – we don't focus on problems, we relax and focus on the solutions instead, the good stuff.

Setting your mind up correctly for relaxation will ensure that you are going to get your subconscious ready for feeding back to you, eventually, the positive images that you want, the positive feelings. Essentially, you are trying to set yourself up for success.

Having this image of the 'doing picture' prior to activating the DMN, really does make sense because this image is what you need to use to nudge your subconscious into the right direction. This is the idea you are presenting to the DMN to work with. If you can get this timing right, if you can get this routine right, this is the secret to emptying your stress bucket.

# The Solution-Focused Formula

S o, in summary, the combination of all these techniques, in a precise order, really does empty your stress
bucket and allow you to begin to feel better quickly. I often
explain to my clients that it is simply a formula. You can
of course use each part of the formula separately and still
notice some benefits. But putting them all together in a
precise way can create real change in the brain.

And the formula is as follows:

◇ What's been good?
◇ Brain basics – revising the brain's anatomy and the
   functions of the intelligent and primitive brain
◇ Scaling and the doing picture
◇ Relaxation; activate the DMN

Begin with 'what's been good', and keep doing that for
a few minutes, taking time to think of as many things as
possible. Then you've done your scaling. On completing
the scaling question, you should have a very clear doing
picture, an image of something that makes you feel good.

If that image does not make you feel good as you read it back to yourself then you may need to start again.

It's important to note also, that image needs detail. The subconscious loves specifics, so make sure your doing picture is something that really makes you feel happy as you imagine it and has the exact details you need; where, when, will anyone else be there? etc.

Don't forget that you are trying to create a positive emotion, you are only using your imagination, so really let your imagination go. This is not a task that you need to ensure that you will do, you are just using your imagination to create a clear, vivid image of what you would be doing tomorrow if you felt a little bit better.

Once you're happy with that image then do your relaxation.

Relaxation is the process of dropping your guard. Remember I said that one characteristic of the primitive brain is vigilance and if you remain vigilant you won't be able to relax. This is training your brain to drop that vigilance.

During relaxation, the primitive brain and the intelligent brain come together and completely relax. When that happens, your DMN gets to work and you can begin to innovate around more positive scenarios and at the same time empty the stress bucket.

Find something that will help you relax. That could be a piece of music, a relaxation or meditation recording, or even some white noise.

Make sure you choose something that you find quite pleasant or unobtrusive because I recommend you stick with this recording all the time and use it regularly, make it repetitive. Every time you hear this recording your mind is used to it. Your mind gets the signal that it is time to relax once again. You need to use something that will not make the mind vigilant so you don't want loud noises and crashes like a heavy drum beat.

This recording only needs to be about 10 to 15 minutes long, not overly long that you may fall asleep to it or find it boring, but also it shouldn't be too short because you need to give yourself time to settle and relax.

Another thing to remember here is to make sure you have something to keep warm like a jumper or even a blanket. When we relax, our body temperature drops and you will start to feel a little bit cooler. If you become too cold it will stop you relaxing, therefore, even if you feel warm at the beginning it's important to still lie under a blanket, so that if you begin to feel cold this doesn't make you more alert and prevent you from relaxing and letting go.

This complete formula of what's been good?, scaling, doing picture and relaxation works by sending a message directly from your intelligent brain to your subconscious.

However, you will be bypassing the primitive brain, you will bypass any negativity and empty your stress bucket.

And really that is all there is to it!

Once you have finished your relaxation carry on with your day as normal.

You don't need to take a long time to do this exercise. The key is repetition, so I recommend you do it once a week.

Within a few weeks you will begin to notice a difference in your mood and mindset and this difference will feel completely natural. You're allowing your subconscious to get to work for your benefit. I often notice changes in clients within one or two sessions. The beauty of solution-focused work is that it can create change quite quickly because we are focusing on future goals, not referencing the past.

Gradually you will find that you have more control over your thoughts and feelings as your stress bucket empties.

Like any other muscle of the body repetition is the key.

Repetition will strengthen that muscle – the brain.

If you would like to, to begin with, you can do this exercise before you go to bed or while you are going on a solitary walk (without your phone!).

It can be a very useful technique to help you sleep, thinking of positive images before you go to bed.

It will help you to relax, focus, and ensure that you are setting your mind up in the correct environment to fall asleep.

## The Bar of Control

I wanted to include a chapter on feelings of control because it's so important to our mental wellbeing.

When people come to see me with an overflowing stress bucket, they have lost control of their thoughts and feelings. They're anxious, stressed and overwhelmed. To get them to feel back in control of themselves and their lives is my aim, and I do this by first of all explaining that control is a good thing.

You will have heard the expression 'control freak' – maybe someone has accused you of being a control freak or you have accused someone of it. Wherever it's been used, it's seen as a negative, something bad, something to be embarrassed about. Well, I'm about to turn that on its head and show you the positive side to feeling in control. I love it when someone calls me a control freak, I take it as a compliment. In fact, I encourage them by saying I'm not a control freak, I'm a control enthusiast (I first heard this from the comedian Sarah Millican and I use it all the time, it's much more solution-focused language, isn't it?).

In solution-focused work we explain that control is a constant, like a bar or a straight line. By this I mean that if you feel in control in one part of your life, you will start to feel in control of many other parts of your life. The key is to focus on the easy stuff first.

You may have heard of the book *Eat That Frog!* by Brian Tracy. It's a fantastic book about how to deal with the big hurdles in life. In summary, Brian explains that if the biggest hurdle you had in the morning was to eat a frog, then you should do that first! You could break it down into pieces or eat it all one go, but either way, eat the frog and get it over and done with. Everything you do after that could never be as bad, you did the worst thing first.

This theory is brilliant and works superbly if you've got an empty stress bucket. I'd encourage you to do that if you're feeling really motivated to.

But if your stress bucket is full the last thing you want to do is eat the frog. When you have a full stress bucket that frog has turned into a massive polar bear and you are in fight-flight-freeze mode! You're consumed by the primitive brain. You will procrastinate and lose motivation, which only increases your anxiety even further.

So, what can you do when you feel like this?

Well, you should take the solution-focused approach and tackle easy, small things first. You know, those simple things you can get under your control, the easy wins, the low-hanging fruit.

For example, if your stress bucket is overflowing then doing something like your tax return may fill you with dread! Brian Tracy would say jump right in and tackle it, break it down, but do this and nothing else. When you've got an overflowing stress bucket though you really can't bring yourself to do it as you are so overwhelmed with your life in general. At the back of your mind, you know it should be done, and you have a deadline, but you feel out of control. Your primitive brain has stepped in to take over. Take a step back from the problem here and focus on a solution. A completely different solution away from the problem itself. What can you get under your control? Maybe it's to tidy up the kitchen, or post those birthday cards you've been meaning to. Shift your focus for a while onto something else. When you do those jobs, you'll feel a whole lot better, your general anxiety will drop and you may then feel you can begin to tackle the tax return.

What you're doing here is slowly coaxing your primitive brain out of its cave by lowering the barriers. You're sort of tempting it to move, just a little, in the right direction of feeling in control, so that you can begin to see that the tax return is not really a polar bear.

This doesn't mean you're procrastinating by doing all the things except that one thing you're supposed to be getting on with. When you lose complete control often you stop doing even all those things you enjoy, the things you find easy, the things that help lower your anxiety. We use this principle all the time in solution-focused work. By focusing on a positive 'doing picture', you are reminding yourself that things can be better, they can improve. You can still achieve things and get them under your control.

**

## *Sarah's story*

Sarah came to see me for generalised social anxiety. However, she had also been having panic attacks, she found driving particularly stressful and had various irrational fears. I had established all this in our initial consultation before sessions began.

Once we got into the swing of our sessions properly though we never spoke once about these fears and anxieties, we focused on what had been good, and what Sarah would do tomorrow if she felt a bit better.

We focused on achievements, raising her self-confidence and self-esteem. It turned out that Sarah was extremely competent in her work of project management. She really enjoyed what she did and could do it with her eyes closed most of the time. When she worked on projects she was in control. We spoke about this a lot, something that Sarah had not really placed much emphasis on previously. Slowly and gradually, she was able to rationalise her fears. Within four sessions Sarah felt much more in control of her thoughts and feelings overall.

During the fifth session, she asked me when we would begin to deal with 'the problem' of driving. As we hadn't mentioned it at all this was totally understandable. I'm sure Sarah even thought that maybe I had forgotten about it. But I explained that we were dealing with it already...by focusing on what she could do and going for the easy wins to help her feel more in control. We were merely keeping it solution focused.

Within a total of six sessions of stress bucket emptying, she was driving with confidence again and her panic attacks stopped completely.

Sarah had been focusing on her problems so much that she had been consumed by them – she thought she needed to analyse why they were present. All she needed to do was feel in control again, and that could only be done by drawing her attention to the things she was good at, the things she could control. If she could easily control those, then, all of a sudden, it seemed easy to control her fear and anxieties as well.

**

What you can control initially may only be small. Things like tidying your sock drawer, or making sure you know what you have for lunch tomorrow may seem trivial, but don't underestimate the power of those small things. Remember you need to gently coax the primitive brain out of its cave.

So, focus on what you CAN control for now. Because slowly and gradually you will be surprised what will appear to feel like it comes under your bar of control.

Due to the fact that I don't talk about problems during sessions, clients often ask me when we will begin to talk about them in a course of sessions – 'when are we going to start dealing with the problem, Gin?' I explain that we already are, by focusing more on the solutions the problems tend to disappear almost as if on their own, and they often wonder why they ever caused a problem in the first place. Taking control is really important. So, go ahead, be a control enthusiast!

Now there are some things that will NEVER be under our control – a lot of people create their own anxiety or stress over these things and fill up their stress bucket unnecessarily. It's really important to remember here that you can't control those actual things but you can control your reaction to them.

I'll give you two examples:

1)   The Weather
You'll never be able to control the weather – it is out of your control. But you can control whether or not you take an umbrella with you, or wear your sunglasses. You can control if you need to make sure you're wrapped up in scarves, gloves and hat, or you can wander about in your flip flops.

2)   Other People
This is a big one. I joke that 'if everyone just did what I said then my life would be amazing!' But it's simply not going to happen, is it? You've got to let go and have some acceptance around this, like you accept the weather. You may not like it but you do have to *accept* it. Having acceptance lowers your anxiety and stress levels considerably.

You can't control other people but you can control your reaction to them. If someone is angry you can choose to engage with them or you can choose to walk away, that is under your control.

If someone is demanding a lot from you, you can choose whether you give in to their demands or to be clear about your personal boundaries.

You have to let go of what you cannot control, it can consume you otherwise. I've seen it consume people and it's not pretty – please think about what is within your control and let go of what isn't, it's really not worth filling up your stress bucket for!

# The Adult–Child Metaphor

It can be confusing to mix metaphors but often I'll see clients that still find it difficult to grasp how irrational the primitive brain is. As a therapist, I don't have a magic wand to fix you, it takes a conscious effort on your part, after all it is your mind and only you can control it.

99% of the time general stress bucket emptying sessions seem to do the trick, but there are a few rare occasions when that primitive brain seems to cling on for dear life and not let go. It can be phenomenally frustrating for me and my clients, and although they understand the principles of what's going on, they need more tools to understand. When this happens, I use the following metaphor to help make sense of it all. It really is a bit of lightbulb moment if nothing has worked so far. I also use this to help people stop smoking.

Imagine your intelligent brain and primitive brain as an adult and a small child respectively. This should make sense as your primitive brain has not evolved or developed, it has remained the same, with a very simple way of looking at things, like a small child. The intelligent brain is developed intellectually, it can rationalise and use lots of objectivity to make sense of things and know why things need to be done, like an adult.

Bear that analogy in mind now as I continue to explain.

A small child (the primitive brain) needs some rules and regulations to keep them safe, yet they are also really clever at knowing how to manipulate adults (the intelligent brain) too.

Imagine one day that you are babysitting for a friend. Your friend tells you their child is not allowed any ice-cream today as they will ruin their appetite, and besides, they've had plenty of treats so far this week anyway. So, armed with that rule, you happily take care of the child for a few hours.

Initially all seems to go well, when gently your charge approaches you and asks for some ice-cream. You say no, as your friend advised and you feel quite sure of yourself. A few moments later maybe the child then looks at you with those huge eyes and a beautiful smile and asks you for ice-cream, they're laying it on thick now! It's harder to resist but you still have your friend's voice ringing in your ears and say no. You feel quite proud of yourself until the child raises their game a little bit more…maybe trying to persuade you with 'please, please, please' or trying to convince you by saying they'll happily share their ice-cream with you – what a temptation!

You find it is becoming more difficult to resist and they really are wearing you down but you stand firm, no ice-cream!

You decide to go to the park to let off a bit of steam. However, children are quite clever, aren't they – they will know that this situation is made for them to get what they want. So, out in public, in front of everyone they decide to throw a tantrum and demand ice-cream! In your embarrassment and panic, you, if you're anything like me when looking after your friends' children, will immediately give in and give them the ice-cream. They win, you lose! Oh dear, you'll be in big trouble with your friend now!

Your primitive brain, like a child, knows exactly what to do and when to convince you to do something you want to stop doing. It can easily throw a tantrum by making you feel you've lost complete control and take you over. It is very clever at presenting you with propaganda to try to convince you to its way of thinking, which you know, intellectually, you're trying to remove yourself from.

It gives rise to sensitive and complex emotions to keep you 'within its grasp' so to speak. It makes you believe that it's too much hard work to resist and easier to give in.

But when you want to break a bad habit, and you know this intuitively, you need to take control from the intelligent brain.

So, let's go back to the adult-child metaphor and make one small, simple change.

Let's say the same thing happens, you have been asked to mind your friend's child and this time there are no rules or regulations set down by your friend. However, after a few minutes of playing at your house the child finds the dishwasher tablets and thinks they are sweets. What would your reaction be now?

The child goes through the whole range of propaganda and manipulation just like before, the big eyes, the pleading, the convincing. I'm sure you would be very strong in saying no, no, no – they are not sweets you are NOT going to eat them.

Even when you go to the park, in public, and they throw the biggest tantrum ever – would you give in then? No way! You, as the adult, know what is best, and you know you'll never let them do that.

In the same way you must take control from the intelligent part of your brain. This is the part of the brain that you know as the real you, the part of the brain that knows what it needs to do to achieve your goals.

And let's face it, would a child behave this way with their own parent, whether it was either ice-cream or dishwasher tablets? Not at all. Boundaries and rules have been set and adhered to. It's not being unkind; you're doing what's best for the child.

In this same way, your primitive brain needs training for its boundaries and rules. Rules set by the much more informed and sophisticated intelligent brain. It's for its own good, even if initially it feels wrong, and it will feel like hard work, you'll be challenged. Long term you will be sure to reap the rewards though.

So, there are two main points to take away from this metaphor when you want to take control from the intelligent brain, the adult.

1) Recognise the propaganda that comes from your primitive brain. What is the language that you use to convince yourself not to do something that you know, deep down, is good for you? What are the signals that come to you? How and when do you give in? Can you pick up on them earlier? Can you try to limit them as much as possible?

2) You need to have a very clear and firm 'No' that comes from the intelligent brain. Drill down into what it is you want to achieve and why it must be done. There should be no argument in your own mind – this is what IS going to happen. No argument!

This metaphor is extremely powerful when trying to create change. Keep it in mind the next time you want to change your way of thinking and create new, positive habits.

When you're trying to create new habits, it's very important to keep solution focused and get some positive emotions behind what you're doing. This method is much more successful than the denial, or problem-focused approach. When people want to change a habit, they only look at the habit itself, or they examine the problem this habit is creating for them. Once you take the solution-focused approach and focus on positive emotions that drive you forward, it becomes so much easier. Initially this takes a bit of work, but this way your habits are much more sustainable, and they don't feel like habits at all, just a way that you live your life.

Using willpower alone does not create new healthy habits, you really need to find some feeling behind it. To do this in a solution-focused way keep asking yourself this one question:

*What would be good about that?*

And don't only do this once or twice – repeat it back to yourself for every answer you give so that you can get to the real emotion behind what it is you want to achieve.

**

## Briony's story

Briony came to see me for weight management sessions. Over the years she had tried many diets but seemed to put the weight back on after a while. She was now in a really successful role at work and the chance of promotion was on the horizon, yet she had little confidence to apply for it, even though she knew she was more than qualified. Her lack of confidence stemmed from the fact that she did not feel presentable due to her weight issues.

We began with general bucket emptying sessions and were making some good progress. Briony's confidence and self-esteem were building gradually, she was sleeping better and feeling happier, but she continued to fall into bad eating habits all the time, something she had been all too familiar with for many years.

I felt that we may stall in progress if not addressed soon because Briony's 'doing picture' always revolved around her weight issues, she was still focused on the problem. Also, her doing picture was often impractical; she would imagine that she would wake up at her ideal weight, or lose a stone overnight – that was not very realistic, it wasn't going to happen so quickly and deep down she knew that.

So, I told her about the adult-child metaphor and what was happening when she needed to take control of her lifestyle habits. We needed to drill down to what was behind the reason she wanted to lose weight, to get that very clear firm 'no' to come from her intelligent brain.

Using the 'what would be good about that?' line of questioning, our conversation went something like this:

Me: I know you want to lose weight, Briony, but what would be good about being your ideal weight?

Briony: Well, I would look good in my clothes.

Me: And *what would be good about* looking good in your clothes?

Briony: I'd be so much more confident.

Me: And *what would be good about* being more confident?

Briony: Lots of things really. I'd be more presentable at work, and deliver my presentations professionally, clearly displaying my knowledge and capabilities, and therefore more likely to get that promotion.

Me: And *what would be good about* getting that promotion?

Briony: Well, what a successful woman I would be – that's the highest rank a female has ever achieved in my organisation.

Me: And *what would be good about* being a successful woman in business?

Briony: I would be setting a wonderful example to my daughters as I want them to grow up feeling like they can achieve anything.

And that was the sweet spot – we'd just hit on Briony's emotion behind WHY she wanted to lose weight. I saw her eyes light up and she realised what all this was about. Surely many people want to lose weight to look good in their clothes, that's a given, but it's not the real reason, is it? And it's still focusing on the problem, bringing to mind that her clothes don't fit well right now. Her real reason was that she wanted to set an example, to be an inspiration to her daughters who she loved. And now she could really see herself doing that.

Once Briony realised this, she was much more motivated to readdress her eating behaviours. Keeping that vision in her mind's eye now meant that addressing her eating behaviours felt right for her, in fact, it didn't even feel like she was doing anything differently, it was the natural way to progress.

Over the next few weeks, the weight seemed to be falling away and even after she had finished sessions, she continued on her weight loss journey. She sent me an email a few months after we had finished sessions – she got that promotion!

**

To really focus in on why you want to do something keep asking yourself, repeatedly, *what would be good about that?* You should be able to easily come up with an answer that will change the way you think completely. Hold onto that as your driving force and refer back to it all of the time. It should only take about four or five repetitions of *what would be good about that?* and you should reach your *why*.

# The Power of Vision

You can spend an inordinate amount of time focusing on all that is wrong with life and knowing what you don't want. But have you ever allowed yourself to focus on what it is you actually want? Have you ever let your imagination go and felt that freedom? Not just dreaming about winning the lottery, but more tangible, positive thoughts about your future?

Once the stress bucket is empty, I help people really focus on this. The brain needs direction, in fact, it can't help being directed. It's your choice whether you want to direct it positively or negatively.

I bet you've heard lots of stories like this: Someone wants to buy a red car, they really have a desire for one, they keep thinking about it, talk about it all the time to their friends and family. Then one day they go on a long journey on the motorway and they spot twenty red cars. Now twenty red cars didn't come out to annoy them, they were always there, other colours of car are there too – but their mind is drawn to only red cars because that's all they've been thinking about.

Maybe it's happened to you. When you want to buy a new house, you see for-sale boards everywhere. When you want to have a child, you see children and babies everywhere. Your mind is drawn to what you focus on.

So, it's time to focus on what you want. And *only* what you want – not what you don't want. (Remember the principle from – DON'T think about a green bus? Keep the talk positive).

The following exercises and considering more long-term visions of your future are much easier when your stress bucket is empty. I often wait till at least six or seven sessions in before I attempt these exercises with my clients. But the results are fantastic.

Let's go back to the happiness scale we use regularly. Number 10 on this scale is the goal you want to reach. However, it's quite natural to move those goal posts regularly and there's nothing wrong with that. Once you empty your stress bucket even a little bit and achieve some goals, you may want to push yourself even further. In a sense, this is what keeps us going in life so stick with it.

But as you get closer to the top, take some time to really think about that number 10. What is the actual goal? If you were number 10 on the scale what would that look like? Can you create a clear, detailed vision of that?

I hope you have realised by now that the imagination is extremely powerful, and the subconscious loves detail, so really take some time to have a clear picture of number 10.

To bring this exercise to life in solution-focused sessions I would ask you to imagine that in about six months' time you are actually number 10 on your scale. Don't get nervous, we're only using your imagination here. Imagine being a 10 and I happen to bump into you in a coffee shop, or I call you up for a chat, and I ask you that question I always ask:

### What's been good?

What would your answer be? What could you tell me about the last six months, if you were now number 10, that would have happened for you to reach that goal? How happy and fulfilled are you?

When you actually role play this in your mind, you'll literally feel your body language begin to change, you'll smile, you'll feel the happiness. The mind doesn't know the difference between imagination and reality, does it?

What this is doing is giving your mind lovely clear direction towards your goals. If you imagine yourself in a new role, then you will be more alert for opportunities. If you imagine yourself being healthier, then you'll be more alert to healthier foods and fitness classes that are around. Just like if you wanted to buy a red car, your mind will bring your attention to what you need in order to achieve that goal. That's the science behind how the brain functions.

I really encourage the role play of this task as it makes it all the more real, but if you can't find someone to help you, or you find it uncomfortable, there is another exercise you could try.

You may have heard of a lot of different versions of writing letters to yourself. It's a really powerful process of accepting things and moving on. However, to stay solution focused about it, try this: write a letter from your future self.

That's right, much like the exercise above, imagine yourself in about six months' time, being at number 10 on your happiness scale and write a letter, as if you were writing a letter to your very best friend, about all the things that have happened over the last six months. In reality you are writing it to yourself but it can help to have someone in mind.

No one is going to see this letter though – it's just something for you. This gives you the freedom to write whatever you want and not have any fear of judgement.

I really recommend writing by hand rather than typing because a lot of creativity will flow this way. Don't worry about your handwriting or your grammar mistakes, it doesn't have to be perfect, simply write in a way that lets your imagination go. Once you begin, you'll be surprised how many ideas and concepts you'll come up with.

You can keep the letter or discard it, it's up to you. Repeat this exercise as often as you wish, maybe every six months or so, as you will naturally move your own goal posts as you keep progressing forward.

Remember, this is just an idea of your vision but do get detailed. It is not a contract set in stone, it's brain training to keep you moving forward positively.

These exercises will enable you to keep focusing on *your* preferred future, and ensure you maintain a positive forward-looking mindset.

Enjoy them and have fun with them, they're not supposed to be a chore, treat them like a bit of a game.

**

I bet by now you're thinking about how full your stress bucket is, how much it's affecting your health, your career, your family, your social life. Maybe you feel it's overflowing, maybe you feel you need a bigger bucket. But if there is one thing you should have learned by reading this book is that you need to be more solution focused. In order to create change you need to stop focusing on the problem.

So, turn it around.

What would your life be like if you had an empty stress bucket?

What difference would that make to your health, your career, your family and your social life? What would be different if you slept better, had more energy and felt positive and motivated every day?

Once you empty your stress bucket you will find more purpose, you will live with more intention. You will be fulfilled.

Believe me when I say, you CAN have an empty stress bucket and, if you can understand the science behind how the brain works, you can keep it empty for life.

# What's been good? – The journal

Take a notebook or use your diary to create positive change in your brain over the course of six weeks with this guide. It should only take you a couple of minutes every day so it's not meant to be a chore but try and fit it into your day somewhere.

This guide should help you get a bit of structure and strengthen neural connections in your intelligent brain, consequently calming down the primitive brain.

What you're going to do is begin the practise of noting down **what's been good** about your day or week and I'm going to help you develop that habit.

As you read the question now it seems surprisingly easy but, on a day when you feel overwhelmed with life and nothing seems to be going right, on a day when your stress bucket is overflowing, it can be a real challenge. It will take a huge amount of effort. But that's when it can make the most difference.

So that's all you are going to make a note of – what's been good.

Only the GOOD things.

Instead of noting down ALL the things that occur, good AND bad, I want you to use your positive filter and only make note of the good things.

These good things do not have to be major events, in fact, I do not expect you to have huge positive events in your life continuously for six weeks, life's just not like that.

The small positive things that you can appreciate are often far more meaningful. And by focusing on them and remembering them, you will create those positive feelings all over again. You may have momentous positive things and that's good too, but you can make a note of absolutely anything that has been good for you.

Things like…

I went for a nice walk.

I had a nice chat with a friend.

I saw a cute dog (my personal favourite!).

Now of course not everything will have been good – that's natural. I don't for one minute deny that you have had stresses and strains. But by focusing on only the good things, you are creating the habit of positive thinking.

You are literally training and rewiring your brain. Engaging the intelligent brain. In turn you can then tackle the issues of life, which we all have, from a more rational perspective. You're using your intelligence to deal with stress rather than your emotion.

## Week 1 – What's Been Good About My Day?

In this first week there will be a task for you to do every single day. This is so you can create the momentum to give you a head start for the following weeks.

You don't have to begin on a Monday. In fact, I would encourage you to begin on any other day of the week *except* Monday.

Mondays generally have quite negative connotations. It's the start of the week and it's a long time till the weekend. So, give yourself a head start by *not* starting on a Monday.

At the end of each day this week I want you to write down three things that have been good about your day – just three. They don't have to be huge, small things will make a difference, it's just appreciation of those good things that happened today.

At the end of the week read back over all the good things that happened. You may have easily forgotten about a good thing that happened earlier in the week, but as you read them back you can relive those positive moments.

## Week 2 – What's been good about my week?

Week 1 got the momentum going – if you wish to continue to note down small, good things every day you can do that. You may even find it helpful as this is not supposed to be a memory game.

However, this week you need to sit down at the end of the week and write a lot more, make a note of as many good things that you can remember.

Small and large, think back over the days and everything you did, and make a note of ONLY the good things.

The key this week is to take your time. Even while you're only trying to think about the good things, you are thinking positively. You are not going towards the negative – only good things.

For ten minutes or so, keep asking yourself, what else has been good about my week…what else…and what else?

**What's been good about my week?**

**Keep going. What else? List as many as you can...**

## Week 3 – Build Your Tribe!

You're doing great so far!

This week you will once again take time at the end of the week to note down all your good things. However, in addition you are going to involve your family and friends in your 'what's been good?' game. You're going to build a tribe of positive people around you.

Instead of asking 'how are you?', I want you to ask friends and family 'what's been good about your day/week?'. Encourage them to talk about their good things, the things that made them happy or some small tasks they achieved.

This can be a great game to play with the family over dinner, encouraging positive talk and therefore positive thinking.

When we create a positive environment around it us it becomes easier to feel positive ourselves.

Once again, note down all the good things about your week. As many as you can, maybe even including things that you enjoyed hearing from family and friends.

**What's been good about my week?**

## Week 4 – Mind Your Language

This week, get detailed about the language you use.

Make sure the language you use is positive when you come to noting down or talking about your good things.

For example, saying 'I didn't feel tired' is not a good thing – reframe that to 'I was full of energy' instead.

Often people will say something negative that they turned into a positive. Although there is some merit in that, you have still given some thought to the negative aspect. That's not really keeping it positive.

For example…

'I had no motivation and felt awful, but I went for a jog anyway and then I felt so energised afterwards.'

By mentioning the fact that you had no motivation, you are thinking negatively. You are recalling a negative memory. Try not to give any thought to the lack of motivation but instead focus on how good you felt after you went for a run.

So, for this week's exercise, make sure you reframe your language to keep it positive and eliminate negative language altogether.

**What's been good about my week?**

_____

_____

_____

_____

_____

_____

_____

_____

## Is my language positive? – If not reframe it here:

## Week 5 – Look To The Future

Continue to note down all the good things about your week.

But now include one or two things you are looking forward to in the future. Maybe you've got a hair appointment booked. Or are meeting a friend for a coffee. Maybe you are looking forward to a great meal that you will have or even going on holiday.

When we feel anxious or depressed, we find it difficult to be forward thinking. Having things to look forward to is what keeps us going in life.

**What's been good about my week?**

**Remember to mind your language.**

**Good things I am looking forward to:**

## Week 6 – Keep Jogging Your Memory, Positively

Continue with this exercise but before you begin to make notes, read back over all of your previous good things. Don't just read them for the sake of it, but take your time to remember them.

I am sure there will be things you had noted in Week 1 that you have forgotten about completely by now. But by going over your good things, you are thinking positively. It will engage the positive, rational and objective part of your brain and help you continue to think about even more 'good things'.

**A good memory from the past is:**

**What's been good about my week?**

_____

_____

_____

_____

_____

_____

_____

**Good things I am looking forward to:**

_____

_____

_____

_____

_____

_____

Well done for thinking positively for six weeks. You did brilliantly.

By now you should feel that you can think positively easily and naturally. So that even in a stressful situation, you can remain objective, rational and in control of your thoughts and feelings.

You will mentally be noting down good things throughout your day, letting them register in the positive part of your brain, exercising and training your mind to focus intelligently.

And you'll be treasuring your positive memories and looking forward to things too.

You will have created a positive tribe around you, encouraging them to think, feel and be more positive.

# To summarise:

◇ Use 'what's been good?' from now on instead of 'how are you?'

◇ Little things count, and are often more important – a cute dog, a nice walk, anything at all – as long as it is a good thing for you.

◇ It will take some effort, consistency and repetition, but remember, you're training your brain.

◇ Take your time. The positive part of your brain takes a bit longer to catch up with you. The negative filter needs to screen first. Silence and pauses to think are fine.

◇ Don't stop – keep asking yourself 'what else?…and what else?'

◇ If someone asks 'how are you?', answer with a good thing and see if it makes a difference to the person you're talking to.

◇ Surround yourself with a positive tribe.

◇ Make it a dinner table game with the family.

◇ You may slip easily into the negative – don't worry about that, it's merely the brain's natural survival response. Keep trying to think of the good things.

◇ Do this regularly – create the habit.

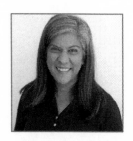

# About the Author

Gin Lalli began her career as an Optometrist and increasingly found that anxiety, stress and depression were having a huge impact on the health and wellbeing of her patients.

She has always been fascinated by how the brain works; why can some people cope with difficult circumstances and others find it more challenging? In order to investigate and understand brain function, Gin began a journey to study neuroscience and psychology, which ultimately led to her becoming a qualified Solution Focused Psychotherapist

She helps people to regain control of their lives by explaining the science behind how the brain functions and by employing the latest evidence-based techniques of positive psychology and neuroscience.

www.ginlalli.com

gin@ginlalli.com

Made in the USA
Columbia, SC
20 September 2023

23138244R00076